Shaping Minds

Discourse Approaches to Politics, Society and Culture (DAPSAC)

The editors invite contributions that investigate political, social and cultural processes from a linguistic/discourse-analytic point of view. The aim is to publish monographs and edited volumes which combine language-based approaches with disciplines concerned essentially with human interaction – disciplines such as political science, international relations, social psychology, social anthropology, sociology, economics, and gender studies.

Volume 32

Shaping Minds. A discourse analysis of Chinese-language community mental health literature
by Guy Ramsay

Shaping Minds

A discourse analysis of Chinese-language community mental health literature

Guy Ramsay
The University of Queensland

John Benjamins Publishing Company
Amsterdam / Philadelphia

The paper used in this publication meets the minimum requirements of American National Standard for Information Sciences – Permanence of Paper for Printed Library Materials, ANSI Z39.48-1984.

Library of Congress Cataloging-in-Publication Data

Ramsay, Guy Malcolm.

Shaping minds : a discourse analysis of Chinese-language community mental health literature / by Guy Ramsay.

p. cm. (Discourse Approaches to Politics, Society and Culture, ISSN 1569-9463 ; v. 32)

Includes bibliographical references and index.

1. Social psychiatry--China. 2. Mental illness--Social aspects--China. 3. Personality and culture--China. I. Title.

RC451.C6R36 2008

362.196'8900951--dc22 2008040161

ISBN 978 90 272 0620 6 (Hb; alk. paper)

John Benjamins Publishing Co. · P.O. Box 36224 · 1020 ME Amsterdam · The Netherlands
John Benjamins North America · P.O. Box 27519 · Philadelphia PA 19118-0519 · USA

This book is dedicated with much love to Sam and Isaac Weier.

Table of contents

Acknowledgements

I wish to thank the following people and organisations for their kind assistance in the development of the Shaping Minds project and the writing of this monograph: Chris Bourke, Ping Chen, Helen Creese, Bai Ding, Yew-Jin Fang, Linda Fleeman, Jill Halil, Obaid Hamid, Wendy Jiang, Asad Khan, Leong Ko, Tony Lai, Wai Wai Lui, Karen Molnar, Polly Nip, Juliana de Nooy, Simon Patton, Veronica Pearson, Judith Ramsay, John Traphagan, Margherita Zanasi, Beijing University Number Six Hospital, Likang Family Resource Centre, Mental Health Association in Taiwan, New South Wales Multicultural Health Communication Service, Queensland Transcultural Mental Health Centre, The University of Queensland, University of Texas at Austin and the reviewers of the monograph manuscript.

CHAPTER 1

Introduction

Mental illness is an affliction widely misunderstood and often feared within societies across the globe. Such fear emerges from its striking at the very core of the human being, the mind. It is the very 'higher order' thought processes and behaviours, deemed to privilege humankind as the supreme life form, which distort or fade when an individual is beset by mental illness. For the person with a mental illness and their loved ones alike the basic tenets of human interactions and relationships, the normative expectations of human growth, development and experience, and the tacit understandings of spiritual being and perceived delineations between spirit and mind are subject to considerable challenge. Certainties of the past no longer hold as understandings of self and identity are reformulated and renegotiated amidst the uncertainties and challenges that accompany the experience of mental illness.

Adding to the mystification that frequently defines the experience of mental illness is the fact that the aetiology of mental illness is often multifactorial and indeterminate, and the prognosis similarly unclear, leaving many people with a mental illness and their loved ones having to come to terms with the prospect of extended and recurring episodes of illness. In such instances, the illness experience often comes to define the life experience, necessitating the seeking and reshaping of new meanings and understandings of one's being. In order to make sense of these changes that mental illness brings, individuals draw on attendant social and cultural resources to interpret the cognitive and behavioural manifestations of the disease and to form judgements as to their aetiological underpinnings. This process of sense making and understanding forms the starting point of this book.

Folk versus biomedical understandings

To state that cultural[1] groups vary in how they view and, indeed, actively construct social phenomena, life experience and notions of fate and providence is rather

1. In this study, culture is defined as per Ting-Toomey (1999, p. 9):

> First, the term culture refers to a diverse pool of knowledge, shared realities, and clustered norms that constitute the learned systems of meanings in a particular society.

trite. Yet this fact is often overlooked in relation to understandings of health and illness. Part of the reason for this arises from the dominance of Western biomedicine in framing such understandings over the last century, which has occurred at an ever-increasing pace with late twentieth century globalisation. Samovar and Porter (2001, pp. 243–244) define biomedicine as a "belief system" that

> focuses on the objective system of diagnosis and scientific explanation of disease … This approach emphasizes biological concerns and is primarily interested in abnormalities in the structure and function of body systems and in the treatment of disease. Adherents … view this model as "real" and significant in contrast to psychological and sociological explanations of illness. Disease is diagnosed when a person's condition is seen as a deviation from clearly established norms based on biomedical science. Treatment through surgery, medicine, or therapy is designed to return the person to the scientifically established "norm."

The subordination of folk understandings of health and illness to those of Western biomedicine amongst public health professionals across the developed and the developing world has seen great advances made in public health. However, sustained improvements in public health necessitate concomitant change in general public beliefs and attitudes. While changing the understandings of health professionals is realized by means of a predominantly Western-premised medical education, changing those of a general public more melded to tradition is significantly more problematic. At the same time, there is a need to consider the desirability of universally supplanting folk beliefs that have evolved from centuries of existence with a biomedical model of Western and, as such, alien origin.

Such issues are of particular salience in the case of mental illness, whose clinical appearance is far removed from that generally conceived of as disease, namely systemic or infectious conditions, and for which a biomedical aetiology has only been established in comparatively recent medical history. Since the clinical appearance of mental illness – the coldness and apathy of depression or the paranoia and deluded thinking of schizophrenia – can easily be misinterpreted as behavioural in nature, it may not be immediately conceived of as pathological in origin. This can delay presentation to health professionals and so worsen the prognosis for the person with a mental illness. In the West, recent decades have seen much effort afforded to public education campaigns seeking to instil a biomedical

---

Second, these learned systems of meaning are shared and transmitted through everyday interactions among members of the cultural group and from one generation to the next. Third, culture facilitates members' capacity to survive and adapt to their external environment.

understanding of mental illness. 'Psychoeducational'[2] formats, such as television and print media advertisements, community awareness weeks and the publishing of informational literature, arguably have seen the biomedical conception of mental illness receive broad community acceptance within the West, at least amongst the non-migrant population.

While psychoeducational campaigns target the community as a whole, they have achieved uneven results across cultural groups in multicultural countries such as Australia and the United States. Here, for instance, there remains significantly lower usage rates of government mental health services and higher involuntary hospital admissions amongst those born overseas, in particular Chinese-speaking migrants, as compared to the locally-born public (Fan & Karnilowicz 2000; Klimidis, et al. 1999a, 1999b; Kung 2001; Loo, Tong & True 1989; Minas, et al. 1996; Sue & Morishima 1982; Tabora & Flaskerud 1997). This occurs despite research showing that the incidence of mental illness remains relatively uniform across cultural groupings (Kleinmann & Mechanic 1981; Leff 1999; Lin, Kleinman & Lin 1981; Steel, McDonald & Hornsey 1995).[3] While access and equity issues may play a role here, such as location of mental health services away from neighbourhoods with high populations of Chinese migrants, a lack of Chinese-speaking staff, along with culturally insensitive or exclusionary institutional practices, ineffective community psychoeducation remains at issue (Bahl 1999; Bhugra, Lippett & Cole 1999; Bhui & Rüdell 2002; Kung 2001; Long, et al. 1999; Sue & Morishima 1982; Yang, et al. 1999).

The biomedical 'normalisation' of mental illness in the West has allowed mainstream recognition of its prevalence within the community, broader discussion of its prevention and treatment, and its inclusion within the greater popularisation of health experienced in recent decades (Gwyn 2002). Yet experiences outside the West and for migrant populations in Western settings remain less clear. While a biomedical understanding of mental illness may prevail amongst health professionals in these contexts, there is a need to determine how such an understanding is being disseminated to the relevant public. Research to date has failed to examine what forms the psychoeducational message takes in such contexts and

2. While the author acknowledges that the expression 'psychoeducational literature', denoting educational leaflets and information sheets produced for the general public on mental health topics, emerges from a biomedical and professional register of usage, this does not by any means indicate a preferred understanding of mental illness by the author. The use of the expression merely reflects the source of the literature under study, namely public health bodies and affiliates, and its continued utilisation throughout the study is purely for convenience.

3. McGrath, et al. (2004), in fact, have documented in migrants a significantly higher incidence of schizophrenia.

how culturally appropriate the disseminated messages may be. It has yet to uncover whether there are differences in the forms of psychoeducational messages presented across cultural settings and, if so, why such differences exist. Exploration of these issues will allow a deeper understanding of how the public health message – here community psychoeducation – is formulated in different cultural settings. It will clarify how a homogeneous view of mental illness based on the biomedical conception embraced by health professionals worldwide is disseminated to heterogeneous populations across the globe. While the intended message may be uniform in relation to content, there is a need to determine the extent to which its discursive presentation varies from setting to setting in order to accommodate the target community. Such enquiry remains of particular importance to multicultural contexts where there exist divergent cultural concerns in relation to mental illness. In such settings are messages formulated differently across resident co-cultures or are the concerns of minority cultures ultimately submerged by those of the dominant culture?

Objectives of the study

This book explores the above issues in relation to a cultural group strongly bound by indigenous traditions, which nevertheless constitutes one of the largest diasporic communities of the Pacific, if not the globe: the Chinese. It will examine how the psychoeducational message is communicated in literature produced across the Chinese diaspora:[4] from the People's Republic of China (hereafter 'mainland China') and Taiwan through to Australia, where Chinese is the most common language spoken after English. The book will explicate differences that emerge in the discursive formulation of the message across the three settings under study. These differences will be examined in relation to the specific contexts of these sites: mainland China as the 'homeland' custodian of traditional culture yet subject to over half a century of authoritarian communist rule; Taiwan as the voice of 'free' China, whose traditions remain unaffected by communist doctrine yet who was subject to 50 years of Japanese colonial rule from 1895 to 1945 and who, since the Allied victory in the Pacific War, has retained strong political and

4. While strictly speaking 'diaspora' denotes communities residing away from their ancestral homeland, for terminological convenience this study employs a broader definition including the People's Republic of China.

cultural ties to the United States; and Australia, whose Chinese communities[5] constitute one of the largest 'minority' cultural groups in an Anglo-dominant society. The salient position of traditional Chinese beliefs will be considered in relation to the three sites under study. Judgements as to the communicative efficacy of the psychoeducational literature from each setting will be made in light of the elicited discursive forms and salient cultural concerns in relation to beliefs and communicative norms.

Communication across cultures

To understand the communication of the psychoeducational message across disparate settings it is necessary to position the phenomenon within the broader context of communication and culture. Communication is culturally determined (Edelstein, Ito & Kepplinger 1989; Garcés 2002; Samovar & Porter 2001, 2003; Ting-Toomey 1999). The manner a message is constructed and presented to an addressee, the deemed appropriateness of linguistic choices employed in the message, the sequence of presentation of ideas and the format adopted to convey the message, amongst other communicative features, are significantly determined by beliefs and expectations held by a cultural group. As Johnson (2003, p. 192) states:

> Culture, then, frames communication by directly influencing its form and content. Routine language use, for example, varies from culture to culture. In this regard … *communicative episodes* … are both highly predictable and culturally specific: Culture provides an individual with shared cognitive schemas that shape language use and broader communicative conduct … Cultural similarity enhances the prospect that language use will lead to communicative effectiveness. Cultural dissimilarity portends the opposite unless cultural mindedness or intercultural communication competence is developed.

This notion of 'intercultural communication competence' is a salient theme in intercultural communication research. The field of intercultural communication studies itself necessarily emphasises the essential connection between culture and communication. Through analysis of communication across diverse cultural communities, research in the field has brought to the light the different ways messages

5. The plural term 'communities' is used here as the Chinese diaspora in Australia has diverse origins, including China, Hong Kong, Indonesia, Malaysia, Papua and New Guinea, Singapore, Taiwan and Vietnam. Chinese-*speaking* migrants, however, are mostly from China, Hong Kong and Taiwan.

are conveyed and constructed, and the significance of this for successful and effective communication. The focus in the main is placed on the 'intercultural' episode whereby people from differing cultural backgrounds engage in communication (Jandt 2004; Ting-Toomey 1999), illustrated in this study by the Australian setting where an Anglo-dominant public health body disseminates a psychoeducational message intended for consumption by a Chinese-speaking readership. However, the 'cross-cultural' enquiry, whereby communicative phenomena are compared across different cultural settings, also falls within this rubric (Jandt 2004; Ting-Toomey 1999). Taken as a whole, this book first and foremost falls under the latter scenario in that the communicative phenomenon of community psychoeducation is compared across three distinct settings: mainland China, Taiwan and Australia. Strictly speaking, the study performs a bicultural analysis (Chinese vs. Australian), given that both mainland China and Taiwan constitute Chinese-dominant societies. However, as already noted in this chapter, the two settings can be distinguished by their disparate socio-political contexts that *may* have a bearing on how public health messages such as community psychoeducational messages are conveyed. Thus, the fundamental principles embodied in the cross-cultural approach remain of relevance to this work.

Another caveat in relation to this study is the hegemonic nature of the discursive genre under study: medical discourse. As discussed earlier in this chapter and forming the central thesis to Chapter 3 of this volume, biomedical understandings of health and illness underpin medical discourse globally. The texts under study here, therefore, are positioned, in actuality, at the interstices of this hegemonic discourse and the cultural forces discussed above. That is to say, while the discursive form of the psychoeducational literature may be subject to and so reflect the cultural context within which it is produced or, more importantly, that of its target audience (as discussed above), at the same time the pervading influence of a biomedical conception of mental illness held by health professionals across the globe may counter this. Thus, potentially, there may be no variance across settings if this hegemonic dominance is all-consuming. The study's data will provide the answer to this question.

The author's earlier cross-cultural studies of Chinese and Australian print mass media text (Ramsay 1997, 2000, 2001a, 2001b) have examined this interrelationship between the discursive form of a 'globalised' text genre and culture. The 1997 study confirmed earlier work by van Dijk (1988) that the essential content presented in news texts from mainland China and Australia, and the global rendering of this content into superstructural schema (namely: HEADLINE – LEAD – BACKGROUND – MAIN EVENT – CONSEQUENCES – EXPECTATIONS & EVALUATIONS), are broadly analogous across cultural settings. However, more local level explication of the news texts' discursive form revealed distinct differences across settings. Specifically, the discursive form of the Chinese texts studied was more digressive; a much lower proportion of main ideas presented in the Chinese texts were realised in prominent positions within their discursive hierarchy; and the Chinese texts placed a greater discursive emphasis on the particulars surrounding reported events, with less emphasis placed on the corroboration and documentation of claims, and on reflection on and questioning of issues (Ramsay 1997, 2000, 2001a, 2001b). Thus, print mass media text, schematically more or less uniform across cultural settings, nevertheless varied significantly in finer aspects of its discursive formulation. The results of the studies suggest that culturally determined discursive styles, such as the preference for inductive rhetoric in Chinese, underpin these differences in what, at least at the schematic level, appears to be a highly uniform text genre.

Variation across cultures even in highly globalised forms of discourse such as print mass media text highlights the importance of considering cultural norms and expectations when constructing a message, given that any mismatch in the rendering of a message can lead to communicative breakdown. There are numerous day-to-day examples of ineffective communication arising from a lack of consideration for or unawareness of culture-bound discursive practices, especially in multicultural social settings. Kirkpatrick (1993, p. 28), for example, cites the following example of a Chinese police constable's (CPC) request for compassionate leave from his British superior (EO) in a Hong Kong police station:

CPC: Sir
EO: Yes, what is it?
CPC: My mother is not very well sir.
EO: So?
CPC: She has to go into hospital sir.
EO: Well, get on with it. What do you want?
CPC: On Thursday sir.
EO: Bloody hell man, what do you want?
(At this point, the police constable mumbled something like 'Nothing sir' and left the office.)

Here, the relatively indirect, delayed presentation of the request for leave made by the Chinese police constable, deemed respectful in light of the seniority of the addressee, on the contrary only serves to irritate his superior. The addressee's cultural expectation in such a context, grounded in his Anglo-British cultural experience, demands a far more direct approach than that being proffered by his subordinate, leading to communicative breakdown. Some understanding on either interlocutor's part of their colleague's cultural expectations in relation to such a communicative act would have avoided the confusion.

The preceding discussion has examined the salience of culture to communication. It has brought to light the relevant elements of intercultural communication theory to this study, noting that where cultures are disparate, that is where "cultural distance"[6] is large, the potential for communicative difficulties is at its highest. This, of course, is of obvious relevance in this study to the Australian setting, where an Anglo-dominant society (and, likewise, its public health institutions) seeks to communicate with a cultural minority (Chinese-speaking migrants). Even when Chinese language is used as the code of communication there remains great potential for the institutional values and communicative norms of the dominant group (Anglo-Australians) to persist in the ensuing discourse, as seen in the Hong Kong Chinese police constable's English-language request for leave.

The discussion has also postulated that differences may equally surface when comparisons are made *across* the settings under study. While cultural distance *per se* may be deemed low when contrasting mainland Chinese and Taiwanese settings (as opposed to mainland Chinese–Australian or Taiwanese–Australian comparisons), both being Chinese-dominant societies, social distinctions such as disparate political histories and outlooks may impact on how mental illness is discursively constructed within each setting. For instance, a blending of traditional Chinese and Marxist conceptions of mental illness may have currency in mainland China, while traditional Chinese, Japanese and American conceptions may be more significant in Taiwan. Such issues are further discussed in Chapter 2 of this volume.

Finally, the preceding discussion has noted that any comparisons need to take into account the hegemony of the biomedical conception of health and illness held by public health bodies globally. This may be expected to attenuate somewhat the extent of difference in discursive form experienced across diasporic settings, although the author's earlier work on print mass media text contests such a view.

Culture and public health communication

How does the relationship between culture and communication translate to the domain of public health communication? Community education is a key element to contemporary public health policy across the globe. Public health bodies deem an informed community to be more likely to engage in healthy life practices, to seek appropriate health care earlier, and to develop greater awareness

6. See Triandis (2003, p. 18) for a definition of "cultural distance" and discussion of the factors contributing to this phenomenon.

and understanding of specific health issues (Arthur 1995; Bhui & Rüdell 2002; Commonwealth Department of Health and Aged Care 1999; Dixon, Adams & Lucksted 2000; Fan & Karnilowicz 2000). This is of particular importance to serious public health issues, such as mental illness. As McCulloch (1998, p. 270) states, a poorly informed public:

> makes life in the community more difficult for people with mental illness … It can affect not only their quality of life, but also their prognosis. And if people are not educated to acknowledge that they or members of their families can become mentally ill, and they are able neither to recognize the symptoms nor to admit their significance, then they will find it difficult to seek help. This results in a huge amount of unnecessary misery and probably in preventable suicides and other negative outcomes.

The "global applicability" of any public health promotion strategy such as community psychoeducation, however, remains problematic given that "'health promotion' is by no means a culture-free entity" (MacDonald 1998, p. 33). Research has emphasised the importance of the adoption of effective and culturally appropriate communicative strategies to the success of community education initiatives addressing serious public health issues (Bhui & Rüdell 2002; Chiu 1987; Garcés 2002; Kuo & Kavanagh 1994; Witte & Morrison 1995). Gallois and Callan (1997, p. 142) have observed that, "It is easy to forget the role of culture in contexts like these, but culture plays a vital role in the success of [public health] campaigns." For example, in relation to HIV/AIDS public education measures in Africa, they have noted the failure of early initiatives to properly take culture into account, with health campaigns unsuitably reflecting "Western cultural values" even though "educators realised early on that cultural values about sexual practice and sex roles would be an important factor in the success of the campaigns" (p. 142). Gallois and Callan have found that recent recognition of the "crucial importance of locally relevant communication" has seen more culturally appropriate community HIV/AIDS education strategies emerge across developing and developed world settings (p. 142). They illustrate as follows (p. 143):

> In most Western cultures, sexual decisions are thought of as the domain of individual people; they are each person's responsibility. Thus, the HIV-prevention campaigns … emphasised individual responsibility. The message was that 'you owe it to yourself to protect yourself from HIV infection' and that 'only you can practice safe sex'. This message is congruent with Western values, in particular the high value put on individualism. It is also compatible with the belief that sex is private and under the control of individual people … The story is quite different in Africa … Here, sexual decision-making is not so private, and is discussed more freely than in most Western countries. On the other hand, many African

> cultures are more collectivist, and place more emphasis on the importance of family life. For these reasons, the Western-driven mass communications fell rather flat in Africa. They were too prudish about sex, and they relied too much on convincing individuals to 'do the right thing'. In more recent years, HIV-prevention campaigns in Africa, and in other communities with similar attitudes and values about sex and the family, have relied more on emphasising a person's obligation to the family ('If you get sick, what will your family do?') … these campaigns have taken a frank and rather humorous approach to sex, something that would probably not be culturally acceptable in many Western countries.

Gallois and Callan's findings neatly demonstrate how consideration of cultural issues can be crucial to efficacious public health communication. Disparate cultures (West vs. Africa) entails disparate communication approaches and styles. The relevance to the current study is clear, that considered attention needs to be given not just to content but to how the intended message is presented when significant belief change is sought, for example, in the case of highly stigmatised illnesses such as HIV/AIDS and mental illness.

'Explanatory models' of health and illness

Through the preceding discussion, it has become apparent that in order to change the prevailing beliefs held by a community in relation to health and illness one first must examine the culture-bound understandings that inform them. As with any social phenomenon, popular "[i]deas about health and illness are grounded in culturally based understandings" (Kuo & Kavanagh 1994, p. 553), and mental illness is no exception (Kung 2001; Williams & Healy 2001). An individual's attempts to make sense of the symptoms and consequences of mental illness, in relation to themselves, a loved one or stranger, will be strongly influenced by how mental illness is conceptualised by society at large. This, in turn, is very much informed by longstanding cultural beliefs (see Chapter 2, this volume). For instance, in Australia the time-honoured belief that depression is simply a transient manifestation of emotional despondency, often suggestive of weakness in personal character, persists amongst some members of the population, leading public health bodies to invest great effort into publicising a biomedical aetiology and pathogenesis for the disease.[7]

---

7. Others may argue that the profits of pharmaceutical manufacturers are also a considerable force here, given that they stand to reap great financial reward from the biomedicalisation of mental illnesses such as depression.

Cultural beliefs are not the sole determinants of an individual's conception of mental illness such as depression – a fundamental premise of this book is that community psychoeducation can lead to belief change – but their salient position should not be underestimated in any public health campaign (Committee on Communication for Behavior Change in the 21st Century 2002). Differences in cultural beliefs, therefore, need to remain "a vital concern … especially … in the realm of health care because diverse cultural experiences produce different expectations and forms of communication" (Samovar & Porter 2001 p. 241). Acknowledging the importance of consideration of cultural nuance and cultural diversity to effective latter-day public health communication, Cora-Bramble and Williams (2000, p. 265) call attention to culturally based "explanatory models for health and illness". A useful concept for this study, explanatory models constitute "beliefs about illness, the personal and social meaning of the illness, expectations about what will happen as a result of illness, how a healer is expected to intervene, and what therapeutic goals are held" (Cora-Bramble & Williams 2000, p. 265). Particularly in multicultural settings such as Australia and the United States, there exists a need to astutely position explanations of health and illness within a target community's broader cultural "framework" or "paradigm" (Cora-Bramble & Williams 2000, p. 265):

> In order to communicate effectively about health and illness, one must understand something about how it is conceptualized and understand aspects of the paradigm in which explanations of health and illness are embedded. Failure to recognize and understand the divergent definitions of illness and conceptions of health will create distance between the health provider and the patient. As the cultural distance increases, so does the likelihood of communication difficulties.

Most effective communication is seen to result when the explanatory models of health and illness held by health professional and health consumer "converge" (Callan & Littlewood 1998, p. 2).[8] Yet, in multicultural settings such as Australia

8. In relation to making sense of mental illness, the concept of "a coherent explanatory model" has been critiqued by Williams and Healy (2001, p. 473), who in a study of "new referrals to a community mental health team" (p. 465) found that in reality individuals "explore and move between a varied and complex set of beliefs … a map of possibilities, which provides a framework for the ongoing process of making sense and seeking meaning" (p. 473). Their study has concluded that "in seeking meaning individuals may hold a variety of explanations simultaneously, or may move rapidly from one belief to another" even after a biomedical cause (psychiatric diagnosis) has been established, and that this exploratory process is not "necessarily problematic to the individual" (p. 473). McCabe and Priebe (2004) have noted the potential fluidity of explanatory models held by people with schizophrenia, with Callan and Littlewood (1998, p. 10) observing in relation to acute psychiatric admissions that "explanatory models can change during the course of a single illness episode". Indeed, these findings are not at odds with the theoretical underpinnings of this study, which, too, acknowledge multiple

and the United States explanatory models often diverge. Despite the best intentions of public health bodies to diminish the communicative 'static' caused by cultural distance, messages these bodies produce, perhaps unwittingly yet ultimately, are colonised by the dominant (Anglo) institutional paradigm. This has a bearing on the communicative efficacy of the public health messages they produce. What is more, professional and lay explanatory models may not necessarily converge even in indigenous settings, for example in relation to mainland China and Taiwan in this study (Kleinman 1980; Phillips, et al. 2000). Here, the biomedical model of health and illness that dominates the health profession globally can diverge significantly from local cultural understandings.

This study, therefore, through analysing community psychoeducational messages propagated in both indigenous and migrant settings across the Chinese diaspora, not only aims to explicate any attendant differences in their discursive forms but also contemplates how the discursive form of a message intersects with local community beliefs ('cultural explanatory models'). As such, any differences observed between professional explanatory model (Chapter 3, this volume) and cultural explanatory model (Chapter 2, this volume) will be considered in relation to achievement of the intended communicative outcome, namely belief change in the direction of the former. In so doing, the potential communicative efficacy of the respective psychoeducational messages will be evaluated.

Shaping minds

This introductory chapter has brought to the fore the fundamental importance of knowledge of and respect for cultural understandings of mental illness for the successful reshaping of community attitudes and beliefs toward mental illness. It has posited that, even though seeking to overcome entrenched popular beliefs, communication of any public health message still needs to be fundamentally culture-centred. This is of particular importance given the highly 'globalised' biomedical understandings of health and illness, including mental illness, held by health professionals across world cultures. It is essential, therefore, to take into

---

extant 'explanations' that may be differentially embraced by individuals (Kleinman 1980). Here, though, it is contended that efficacious, culturally appropriate psychoeducation can instil a deemed preferred belief amongst the *broader community*. While community beliefs will to a significant extent inform those held by people with a mental illness, the author acknowledges the extra considerations impacting on this group, so that claims made in this study of community psychoeducation are necessarily more equivocal in relation to the psychoeducational experience of *people with a mental illness*.

consideration the potential discord between the message intended for communication by the public health body and the cultural understandings of the target community if effective psychoeducation is to take place. Such consideration is necessary in both indigenous contexts and where the target community is of migrant origin, although the potential for miscommunication is likely to be greater in the latter case, given that, as Johnson (2003, p. 192) states, "In a multicultural society, there is plenty of room for communicative misunderstanding and conflict based on different language systems, which arise from different cultural systems and their accompanying discourses."

Chapter 2 of this volume discusses the cultural conceptions of mental illness (cultural explanatory models) salient to the Chinese societies under study. It documents these conceptions from imperial times through to present-day, encompassing traditional Confucian, religious and medical understandings along with literary portrayals of the times. The chapter examines the impact of Western scientific and political ideas imported during the twentieth century on conceptions of mental illness, in both republican and communist era China and Taiwan. The essential challenges cultural explanatory models and culture-bound stigma present to community psychoeducational strategies emerge from this discussion.

Chinese health professionals would be expected to have insight into indigenous cultural explanatory models, yet their own understanding will be strongly conditioned by the professional explanatory models gained during their medical training. Their cultural understanding or "*primary discourse*: that discourse "to which people are apprenticed early in life"" to a marked extent will be subsumed by professional understandings or "secondary" discourse: that which people acquire later in life "[a]s members of groups" [original emphasis] (Johnson 2003, p. 192). Chapter Three of this volume, accordingly, turns to the setting within which the psychoeducational message is constructed, exploring the discursive underpinnings of the contemporary medical experience of health and illness. The chapter firstly presents a discourse analytic model to frame this study, discourse analysis being a disparate, multidisciplinary field of research. The model framing this study postulates an inter-positioning, in communicative undertakings, of discourses, as ways of representing aspects of the world; texts, as tracts of language in use; and social experience. Moreover, an intersection and blending of multiple discourses, in both synergic and antagonistic associations, sees discursive hybridity characterise most communicative events.

Chapter 3 also documents the distinctive ways the medical profession represents health and illness, particularly mental illness and mental health care. The means by which this professional outlook is promulgated in communicative undertakings, be they doctor-patient interviews, clinical rounds or, as of concern here, public health educational texts, is brought to light. The chapter reviews earlier discourse analytic research on medical discourse and elucidates a hybrid construct variably resonating three salient 'voices': the professional, privileging specialised practice and expert knowledge; the institutional, privileging the established organisational structure and the maintenance and assertion of a hegemonic position; and the client-centred, a recently emerging counter-discourse privileging life experience and consumer empowerment (Ramsay 2004a). Within this conceptual framework, any instance of medical communication will embody these discursive forms to a greater or lesser extent. Moreover, determination of dominant discursive forms, their intersections and articulations provides insight into the intended communicative outcome and its manner of propagation.

Chapter 4 of this volume describes the discourse analytic framework employed in the study and its application to the literature of concern. The Rhetorical Structure Theory (RST) framework, as applied in the author's earlier research (1997, 2000, 2001a, 2001b), is used to explicate the discursive form of the psychoeducational literature sourced from across the Chinese diaspora. Drawing on the notion of medical discourse as a hybrid construct, as discussed in Chapter 3, results obtained from the RST analysis allow determinations to be made as to the degree of resonance of professional, institutional and client-centred voices within each regional corpus of psychoeducational literature. Based on the model of discourse analysis framing the study, this chapter, therefore, examines the inter-positioning of text and discursive practice. The inter-positioning of text, discursive and social practice is explored in Chapter 5.

In Chapter 5, the significance of the findings from the preceding chapter for each regional corpus of psychoeducational literature is discussed, subsequent to evaluation of the potential communicative efficacy of the literature for effecting intended belief change in the target communities. Comparisons are made of the discursive strategies evident in the psychoeducational literature from each of the diasporic regions. Differences observed are discussed in relation to the deemed proclivity of certain discursive forms to facilitate belief change in the target community, given prevailing cultural explanatory models, as documented in Chapter 2. Thus, for each regional corpus, comments are made as to the significance of and reasons for the presence of specific discursive features in their psychoeducational texts, both as a group and individually; and judgements are made as to the appropriateness of the discursive makeup of the psychoeducational message in light of the cultural explanatory models informing the beliefs deemed to require change. The relevance of these findings to public health bodies across the global Chinese diaspora is considered.

In the concluding chapter, Chapter 6, the issues raised in this introductory chapter are revisited in light of the findings produced by the study. New insights gained into community psychoeducation in indigenous and migrant settings, and in relation to medical discourse more broadly, are discussed, along with the attendant theoretical implications for this study's guiding disciplines: discourse analysis, cross-cultural communication and health communication.

CHAPTER 2

Chinese cultural explanatory models of mental illness

The previous chapter has brought to light the importance of culture to people's conceptions and understandings of mental illness. As a formative influence from birth, culture, or its mediated experience within the contexts of family and broader society, strongly dictates how people come to think about departures from what is commonly deemed normal in a society, be it in relation to behavioural conduct, disability or illness. Unless a credible, accessible alternative is presented to an individual, culturally determined conceptions of difference will continue to preside. Hence the importance of community psychoeducation, in the case of mental illness, in disseminating new conceptions of mental illness that are plausible in light of widely held beliefs and knowledge and, as such, able to replace, or at least challenge to a significant extent, culturally determined understandings and meanings.

In seeking to explicate the discursive form of Chinese-language psychoeducational literature drawn from three diasporic settings, the need to understand the cultural and socio-pragmatic contexts from within which the literature emerges is crucial to this study. One cannot successfully make sense of the existence of particular discursive positionings in the case of community psychoeducation unless one fully grasps the cultural context within which psychoeducation resides, facets of which it may seek to counter (Schiffrin 1994). As noted in Chapter 1 of this volume, the limited initial success of community HIV/AIDS campaigns on the African continent can be explained in part by public health educators overlooking the pivotal role of culture (Gallois & Callan 1997). Before analysing the discursive forms of the psychoeducational literature under study, this chapter, therefore, will document the salient cultural understandings and beliefs pertaining to mental illness found in Chinese societies from traditional through to contemporary times. In so doing, the formative influences on lay and professional conceptions of mental illness and what this means for community psychoeducation across the present-day Chinese diaspora will be evaluated.

The chapter firstly determines what the dominant explanatory models of mental illness were in traditional Chinese times, from the early imperial period up to the early twentieth century when civilian rule began (1912). Folk and traditional medical conceptions of mental illness are described and their potential impact on lay explanatory models along with their contribution to Chinese cultural stigma toward mental illness is discussed. The influence of the dissemination of Western knowledge and theories during the modern period (1912–1949), at least among the elites of republican Chinese society, is then considered. The situation is re-evaluated through the contemporary period, which follows the communist victory on the mainland in 1949. This period saw communist orthodoxy dominate mainland China until the economic reform period (1978 to date), when a greater focus on both Chinese tradition and Western ideas has re-emerged. In Taiwan, on the other hand, an exiled republican government and successive administrations, strongly allied to the United States, have presided over a Chinese society where cultural values and norms have remained for the most part unchallenged by antithetical ideologies. The impact of these divergent contemporary experiences on how members of the respective communities conceptualise mental illness and, additionally, how members of these communities who emigrate negotiate understandings in their 'host' destinations, are addressed.

Traditional conceptions of mental illness in China

In seeking to understand contemporary lay thinking about mental illness it is useful to examine traditional understandings of mind, illness and mental illness, which may have informed the existing views prevailing in Chinese societies (Lin, Tseng & Yeh 1995). In the dominant teaching of Chinese culture, Confucianism, notions of the 'mind' entailed the definitively human feelings of "commiseration (benevolence) … shame and disgust (righteousness) … humility and consideration (propriety) and the sense of right and wrong (moral judgment)" (Tseng 1973a, p. 193). These correspond to the venerated Confucian qualities of *ren* (仁), *yi* (义), *li* (礼) and *de* (德), respectively. Loss of mind, therefore, saw the individual 'disembodied', losing "the ability to function not only as a social, but as a cultural entity" and becoming "burdensome and embarrassing to the most immediate group to which he belongs – the household" (Traphagan 2000, pp. 8, 153). Moreover, the consequences of this disembodiment extended beyond the immediate context of the family to broader society, the nation and afar:

> when the mind is purified, then one can cultivate his moral character; when he has cultivated himself, he can head his own family successfully; when he is head of the family, he can serve and regulate his own country; when he can serve the country, then he can attain the final goal of serving the world by his virtue.
>
> (*Great Learning*, 大学, cited in Tseng 1973a, p. 193)

Loss of mind, therefore, portended serious consequences in traditional Chinese thinking, fundamentally threatening notions of order and harmony that lie at the core of Confucian teachings (King & Bond 1985; Kung 2001; Lin, Tseng & Yeh 1995; Metzger 1981). Loss of mind also threatened the core Confucian precept of maintenance of the family line through male heirs. Patrilineal continuity demanded production of *healthy* male offspring:

> Patrilineal culture, in which reproduction was represented as something potentially dangerous that should be carefully regulated in order to safeguard the lineage's future, permeated many medical publications in the late imperial period. Individuals were represented as a key element in a patrilineal line of descent, envisaged as an indispensable link connecting past ancestors and future descendents, and as such were enjoined to regulate and administer their reproductive behaviour for the sake of the lineage. The individual, seen in relationship to the lineage, was held to be responsible not only for his or her own reproductive behaviour, but also for the health of future offspring. (Dikötter 1998, p. 8)

Mental illness presented a clear threat to the preservation of healthy future generations as its hereditary potential was well recognised in Chinese culture from early on (Lin 1981; Ran, et al. 2005).

The challenge mental illness presented to these deep-seated traditional values explains the acute stigma toward mental illness that is widely acknowledged to permeate Chinese societies, both past and present (Bahl 1999; Bentelspacher, Chitran & Rahman 1994; Fan & Karnilowicz 2000; Loo, Tong & True 1989; Phillips 1993; Ran, et al. 2005). Pearson (1996, p. 438) states:

> Of all conditions, mental illness is one that confounds a culture that values conformity, discretion, modesty, and rectitude. The potential for disorder and nonconformity that severe mental disorder represents – particularly the symptoms of mania and schizophrenia – is deeply disturbing within Chinese society. Stigma and rejection of the mentally ill are common experiences in most societies, but in China they seem to be felt with a particular intensity.

When mental illness occurred the burden on the family in imperial China was great. Not only did family members need to deal with the hurdle mental illness presented in meeting Confucian ancestral duties and an attendant loss of 'face', but they also had to cope with rejection from society at large. Moreover, in imperial times immediate responsibility for care of people with a mental illness remained with the family. This reflects the central role of family in Confucian societies. Chiu (1981, p. 81) notes that early in the Qing rule (1644–1911):

> a sub-statute was enacted, spelling out clearly the obligations of relatives, community, and officials. Relatives were given the initial duty to report the existence

> of an insane family member and keep him in strict confinement. If the family failed to report to the authorities or the insane had no family, then neighbors, clan heads, and local leaders were explicitly instructed to take charge. The district magistrate was expected to exert verbal pressure by ordering the family and the like to keep the insane under strict surveillance. To top it all off, any one who neglected to do his part, resulting in the insane killing himself or others, was subject to specified penalties.

Such reporting provisions conflicted with one's Confucian duty to patrilineal continuity and filial piety, which saw families extremely reluctant to publicly divulge the existence of mental illness in the family (Chiu 1981). Revelations were considered shameful, in all likelihood to lead to family members being excluded from the marital pool, and filially inappropriate where parents or elders were suffering from mental illness. In most cases people with a mental illness simply were hidden away from the community, usually detained within a room in the family home and often shackled (Chiu 1981). Only the most severely disturbed acutely psychotic individuals were incarcerated by the state, usually dangerous forensic cases involving serious crime such as homicide (Chiu 1981).

Historical practice in China through imperial times and well into the modern (republican) period rarely saw people with a mental illness institutionalised (Pearson 1996; Ran, et al. 2005). Asylums for the insane did not appear in China until the turn of the twentieth century, under the tutelage of Western missionaries (Hsueh-Shih 1995; Kleinman 1986; Pearson 1996; Ran, et al. 2005; Tseng 1986). Families, therefore, determined the form of care, if any, that people with a mental illness received. Help-seeking responses were determined by the cultural explanatory model that families subscribed to. For the vast majority of the lay population in imperial times, poor and illiterate, mental illness was viewed as spirit or demonic possession or retribution for ancestral misdeeds. The primary avenue for care was folk healers (Li & Phillips 1990; Tan 1981; Unschuld 1985).

The link between the supernatural and mental illness, in particular psychosis, is commonly recounted in traditional fiction, such as *Strange Stories from a Chinese Studio* (聊斋志异), an eighteenth century anthology of supernatural tales written by Pu Songling (蒲松龄):

> A certain mad priest, whose name I do not know, lived in a temple on the hills. He would sing and cry by turns, without any apparent reason; and once somebody saw him boiling a stone for his dinner. At the autumn festival on the 9th day of the 9th moon, an official of the district went up in that direction for the usual picnic, taking with him his chair and his red umbrella. After luncheon he was passing by the temple, and had hardly reached the door, when out rushed the priest, barefooted and ragged, and, himself opening a yellow umbrella, cried

> out as the attendants of a mandarin do when ordering the people to stand back. He then approached the official, and made as though he were jesting at him; at which the latter was extremely indignant, and bade his servants drive the priest away. The priest moved off with the servants after him, and in another moment had thrown down his yellow umbrella, which split into a number of pieces, each piece changing immediately into a falcon, and flying about in all directions. The umbrella handle became a huge serpent, with red scales and glaring eyes
> (Pu 1916, p. 426).

Ng (1990) interestingly observes that in traditional Chinese society spirit possession as a cause of mental illness may actually have been less stigmatised than ancestral transgression, as the former can be considered more indiscriminate in nature, a consequence of ill fortune rather than familial shortcoming. On the other hand, a seemingly chance possession of an individual could still in the end be attributed to fundamental vulnerabilities in the individual concerned and accordingly re-accentuate the familial connection and its associated stigma.

In imperial times, Traditional Chinese Medicine (TCM) provided alternative understandings of mental illness to the folk models described above. TCM's holistic approach to illness views interaction between the natural environment and the body and its affect on organ homeostasis within the body as accounting for disorders in health, including those known as mental illnesses today (Chiu 1986; Leung 1998). Disease of the mind *per se* was not broadly distinguished, with the aetiology of emotional and behavioural symptomatology generally attributed to underlying problems afflicting organ systems in the body. For instance, TCM viewed happiness as coupled to the heart, anger as coupled to the liver, worry as coupled to the lungs, fear as coupled to the kidneys and desire as coupled to the spleen (Lin 1985). Emotional and behavioural disturbances were believed to originate from imbalance or disharmony, resonant of the Confucian social tradition, in the complementary Taoist elements *yin* (阴) and *yang* (阳), in the flow of the universal life force *qi* (气) or in the status of "a person's vital energy" *jing* (精), (Chiu 1986, p. 37). In contrast to folk beliefs, in TCM spiritual and demonistic aetiologies for the most part were de-emphasised, although greater reference to these aetiologies in TCM texts occurred during the high point of religious (Taoist and Buddhist) influence leading up to and including some years of the Tang dynasty (618–907) (Tseng 1973b). This subsequently declined with the re-assertion of Confucianism during ensuing dynasties (Ng 1990; Tseng 1973b).

The somatisation or "normative expression of personal and social distress in an idiom of bodily complaints and medical help-seeking" (Kleinman 1986, p. 2) that characterises TCM saw few explicit references made to depressive illness in TCM until Ming times (1368–1644), while depression was well recognised in ancient Greece (Kleinman 1986; Tseng 1973b).[1] At the time, Wang Kentang (王肯堂, 1549–1613) formally proposed an explicit higher-order category of mental illness in TCM, *shenzhi* (神志), marking "a landmark in the history of Chinese psychiatry" (Chiu 1986, p. 45). This categorisation, however, failed to impact on later imperial-period medical texts, indicating that explicit higher-order classification of mental illness "always remained only a minor strand in Chinese medical thought" (Chiu 1986, p. 300). This subordination, Lin (1985, p. 386) states, "exerted an inhibiting effect on the development of psychiatry as an independent system of psychological medicine as it is in the West" and saw depression remain broadly unrecognised clinically until very recent times.

While TCM explanatory models for the most part somatise mental illness, it is believed that the somatic presentation of mental illness that characterises Chinese societies can also be attributed to the aforementioned deep-seated cultural stigma against mental illness (Cheung 1995; Chiu 1986, Kleinman 1986; Kua, Chew & Ko 1993; Lin 1985). Somatisation allows an "ambiguity of expression about mental distress without bearing the stigma of psychiatric illness" (Cheung 1995, p. 162). Responses to physical illness are relatively straightforward, merely entailing the acquiring of appropriate remedies provided by TCM or folk medicine. Treatment of mental illness, however, is much more problematic due to the nature of its aetiological basis, such as spirit possession and heredity, and the sensitivities that accompany such conceptions. Kleinman (1986, pp. 54–55) believes that stigma along with allied cultural norms predispose Chinese people to somatise mental disorders:

> culturally shaped psychological processes lead Chinese to suppress distressing emotions. These processes include valuing the harmony of social relations over the expression of potentially disruptive and ego-centered intrapsychic experience; a situation orientation that emphasizes state appropriate emotional expressions over trait appropriate ones; cognitive coping mechanisms that systematically employ externalizing idioms of distress over internalizing ones; strongly negative valuation of the open verbal expression of personal distress outside close family relations, which is viewed as embarrassing and shameful; the use of a rich cultural code of bodily metaphors of psychosocial problems; and a desire to avoid the strong stigma that attaches to families with members labelled emotionally ill … These and other traditional cultural concepts and norms … overdetermine a somatic idiom for the expression of personal and social distress among Chinese.

1. Kleinman (1986, p. 56) argues that "from the cross-cultural perspective it is not somatization in China (and the West) but psychologization in the West that is unusual and requires explanation."

Nevertheless, there remains an important exception to the somatisation of mental illness, namely schizophrenia and related psychoses, whose pathogenesis in TCM has always been associated with dysfunction of the mind (Chiu 1986). This conception of the pathogenesis of psychosis provides evidence for Chiu's (1986, p. 302) claim that, despite the supremacy of the paradigm of integration between mind and body, TCM still retained "a mode of discourse which expresses mental symptoms in direct, specific language." Reference to psychotic forms of madness or *kuang* (狂), in fact, dates back to the *Huangdi Neijing* (皇帝内经), a seminal ancient Chinese medical text most likely originating from the Han Dynasty (206BC-220AD) (Chiu 1986; Hsueh-Shih 1995; Ng 1990; Tseng 1973b). Recommended therapy at the time essentially comprised non-intervention:

> If a patient wants to go, let him go; if he wants to stay, let him stay; do not deny him what he wants and do not suppress him. If we comply to his wishes and let him satisfy his needs, then all of his excessive positive force will be appropriately discharged and he will consequently get well. (Tseng 1973b, p. 571)

In later imperial times herbs came to form the basis of treatment of psychosis (Tseng 1973b).

While in TCM the pathogenesis of psychosis (largely emanating from the mind) was differentiated to some extent from that of the somatised mental disorders such as depression (largely emanating from the body), Lin (1985, p. 386) claims that the pervasiveness of somatisation in the Chinese illness experience and the high incidence of paranoid symptomatology found in Chinese people suffering from psychosis, nevertheless, both embody a "turning away from intrapsychic mechanism – the former through bodily manifestation, and the latter projecting to person(s) or happenings in the outside world." In other words, whether suffering from somatised depression or psychosis, for the individual concerned the root cause of illness is similarly located beyond their minds. Such rationalisation may allow for maintenance of a semblance of 'face' for the individual concerned.

In sum, in TCM it appears that the supremacy of a paradigm of integration between mind and body saw only the most unmistakably (i.e., socially disruptive) psychological pathology, such as psychosis, conceptualised as a higher-order mental syndrome. This singular distinction of psychosis as disease of the mind would have only added to its social stigmatisation. It is important to note, however, that in imperial times the vast majority of lay Chinese did not possess the financial means to access qualified practitioners of TCM. Its role in influencing lay explanatory models of mental illness remains unclear. Nevertheless, the fundamental beliefs of TCM and its attendant conceptions of mental illness provided a framework of understanding for some.

The conceptions of mental illness salient to traditional Chinese society documented so far in this chapter neatly accord with Unschuld's (1985, p. 7) taxonomy of Chinese aetiological schema for illness more broadly:

1. The Paradigm of Cause-and-Effect Relations between Corresponding Phenomena
    - 1.1 Causation through Magic Correspondence
        - 1.1.1 Homeopathic Magic
        - 1.1.2 Contact Magic
    - 1.2 Causation through Systematic Correspondence
        - 1.2.1 Yinyang Correspondence
        - 1.2.2 Five Phases Correspondence
2. The Paradigm of Cause-and-Effect Relations between Noncorresponding Phenomena
    - 2.1 Causation through Intervention by Supranatural Phenomena
        - 2.1.1 Ancestors
        - 2.1.2 Spirits and Demons
        - 2.1.3 God(s)
        - 2.1.4 Transcendental Law
    - 2.2 Causation through Influence of Natural Phenomena
        - 2.2.1 Foods, Drinks
        - 2.2.2 Air, Wind
        - 2.2.3 Snow, Moisture
        - 2.2.4 Heat, Cold
        - 2.2.5 Subtle Matter Influences
        - 2.2.6 Parasites, Viruses, Bacteria, and others.

Categories 1.1 and 2.1 encompass lay mystical and spiritual understandings dating back to early imperial times. Categories 1.2 and 2.2.1–2.2.5 encompasses TCM conceptions, while category 2.2.6 encompasses those of Western medicine, which, while disseminated throughout China by Western missionaries in the nineteenth century, came to prominence in China in the twentieth century (Unschuld 1985). These aetiological conceptions along with other relevant Western ideas that came to prominence in the twentieth century are discussed in the following sections.

Conceptions of mental illness in modern China (1912–1949)

The fall of the Qing Dynasty in 1911 saw great changes in China socially and politically. While Western ideas were already receiving greater prominence in the latter period of Qing rule as overseas trained scholars returned to China, the late 1910s and 1920s saw a dramatic movement against Confucian traditions and supporting 'modernisation'. By the 1930s, the embracing of Western scientific ideas made possible the appearance in China of the study and practice of psychiatry (Hsueh-Shih 1995; Kleinman 1986; Pearson 1991). While remaining embryonic in the modern period and concentrated in the major urban centres, this development of psychiatry set the stage for a greater expansion in decades to follow. For the most part, the experience of these social changes of the modern (republican) period was limited to the urban intellectual elites of major centres such as Shanghai and Beijing. Communism with its anti-traditionalist revolutionary stance and strong attraction to the Western scientific tradition, however, ultimately was disseminated much more widely across China, leading to a decisive victory for the communists in 1949.

As in imperial times, mental illness, notably psychosis, featured as a recurring theme in popular fiction. Many modern authors allegorically framed iconoclastic attacks on the traditions deemed to maintain the inequalities and injustices of Chinese society at this time through representations of madness. The first and arguably most important work of modern fiction, Lu Xun's (鲁迅) *Diary of a Madman* (狂人日记), published in 1918, recounts the paranoid delusions of a young man with schizophrenia who fears society is literally seeking to devour him and who only regains his sanity through his eventual "collaboration with the established order" of Chinese tradition (McDougall & Louie 1997, pp. 94–95). In the following excerpt curious locals observe the 'madman' in his home:

> Outside the gate stood a group of people, including Mr. Chao and his dog, all craning their necks to peer in. I could not see all their faces, for they seemed to be masked in cloths; some of them looked pale and ghastly still, concealing their laughter. I knew they were one band, all eaters of human flesh. But I also knew that they did not all think alike by any means. Some of them thought that since it had always been so, men should be eaten. Some of them knew that they should not eat men, but still wanted to; and they were afraid people might discover their secret; thus when they heard me they became angry, but they still smiled their cynical, tight-lipped smile.
>
> Suddenly my brother looked furious, and shouted in a loud voice:
>
> "Get out of here, all of you! What is the point of looking at a madman?"
>
> Then I realized part of their cunning. They would never be willing to change their stand, and their plans were all laid; they had stigmatized me as a madman. In future when I was eaten, not only would there be no trouble, but people would

> probably be grateful to them. When our tenant spoke of the villagers eating a bad character, it was exactly the same device. This is their old trick.
>
> (Lu 1972, pp. 16–17)

Attitudes toward mental illness amongst the intellectual and governing elites of the modern period were further evident in the "eugenic vision" of 1920s and 1930s China, "a period of drastic political, social and cultural change during which ideas of racial hygiene permeated almost every field related to human reproduction, from birth control to sex education" (Dikötter 1998, p. 3). In response to the standing of the eugenic vision in the West at this time, many in Chinese scientific and government circles embraced a notion that promoted the need to strengthen the quality and resilience of the Chinese gene pool by eliminating the deemed imperfect or inferior. This occurred despite more extremist proposals in China, as Dikötter (1998, p. 112) notes, "for eugenic laboratories at the provincial level and special villages, where people with perfect brains and ideal bodies could be bred in order to generate the future 'model race'", along with "plans for the 'forcible elimination' of entire categories of people judged deficient", which included the "mentally disordered."

Dikötter (1998) argues that the Chinese eugenic vision, which, as will be seen, maintains currency in contemporary reproductive discourse promulgated by the communist state, merely reconstituted the traditional Chinese cultural emphasis on patrilineal continuity that commanded the production of healthy male offspring to continue one's family line. Here, scientific rationale was enlisted to legitimise longstanding cultural beliefs, including those discussed earlier which traditionally marginalised people with a mental illness. As a consequence, the eugenic vision reinforced the serious stigma attached to families with a history of mental illness by "collud[ing] with patrilineal culture, in particular folk models of inheritance which see disorders as running in family lines" (Dikötter 1998, p. 181).

The penetration of the eugenic vision across all echelons of Chinese society of the time, in particular the vast rural poor, would have been limited. Education and literacy levels in the countryside were low, few had access to the mass media and dialect-based language barriers across China were considerable. However, the significance of the popularisation of the eugenic vision amongst the elites of modern China lies in the fact that there remained no challenge to the negative conceptions of mental illness that characterised traditional times. These conceptions in fact retained currency in the modern period particularly among the rural masses and, as elaborated in the following section, still retain varying degrees of influence today (Unschuld 1985).

Conceptions of mental illness in contemporary China and Taiwan (post-1949)

Two distinct 'indigenous' Chinese societies emerged from the communist victory in the Chinese Civil War in October 1949: one on mainland China and the other on the neighbouring island of Taiwan. Each was governed by quite disparate political systems, which led, in many respects, to differing social outlooks and practices. Until the death of veteran communist leader Mao Zedong in 1976, 'cross-straits' differences were marked, with mainland China following doctrinaire communism while Taiwan continued to attach great importance to the Chinese Confucian tradition at the same time looking westward to the United States for security. Since the 'open door' liberal economic reforms introduced on the mainland in 1978 by paramount Chinese leader Deng Xiaoping, cross-straits differences in many areas have become less marked with both societies focussed on developing Western-style modernisation programs and expanding the market economy. Nevertheless, cross-straits tensions remain high with mainland China hostile to Taiwan's recent contemplations over independence (Taiwan remains a renegade province of China in the eyes of most of the world) and with many regional democratic states, such as Australia, more supportive of China in the international theatre as a consequence of China's position as a regional economic power.

China

The development of psychiatry that occurred in China during the modern period continued into the contemporary period. Mental health services expanded after the communist victory in 1949, with Soviet neuropsychiatry dominating psychiatric practice through the 1950s and 1960s, although the emphasis on the individual that underpins psychiatry remained of continuing concern to the political authorities of the time (Kleinman 1986; Pearson 1996; Ran, et al. 2005; Tseng 1986; Yan 1985). Such suspicion saw the provision of mental health services severely disrupted during the Cultural Revolution (1966–1976), a chaotic decade where leftist political ideology dominated and mental illness was seen more as a subversive manifestation of incorrect political thought (Boey 1997; Hsueh-Shih 1995; Kleinman 1986; Ran, et al. 2005; Tseng 1986; Xia & Zhang 1981). Post-Mao China has experienced significant expansion in hospital and community based mental health services and in the practice and study of contemporary psychiatry (Ran, et al. 2005). A Western-based biomedical approach to mental illness now dominates contemporary psychiatric practice in China, with possible vestiges of the somatic elements of traditional Chinese medicine (Kleinman 1986; Pearson 1995b; Phillips 1993; Ran, et al. 2005; Tseng 1986).

As was the case in imperial times, families in contemporary China remain ultimately responsible for monitoring people with a mental illness and ensuring that they do not disrupt social order (Ran, et al. 2005). Over ninety percent of people with chronic schizophrenia in China live at home with their families, considerably higher than the corresponding figure for the United States, only forty percent (Phillips 1993; Ran, et al. 2005). This places a particular burden on the families given that eighty percent of people with a serious mental illness still remain untreated in China (Pearson 1996; Ran, et al. 2005). According to Ran, et al. (2005, p. 8), reasons for this high percentage of untreated include: "Poor recognition of mental illness, stigmatization associated with psychiatric illness, family low-economic status [particularly in rural and remote areas], and lack of trust in psychiatric services." The high level of untreated, unfortunately, continues to see the physical restraint of people with a mental illness by their families in present-day China (Pearson 1996). In many cases, hospital care is only sought when the burden of home care becomes too great for the family, when public disturbances occur or when family caregivers die (Pearson 1995c). Effective community psychoeducation would go a long way in addressing many of these issues. Indeed, Pearson (1996, p. 450) has found that mainland Chinese families caring for family members with a mental illness "show a desire to know more about the illness and how to handle th[e] patient best at home", with families often quite unsatisfactorily having to "glean the scraps of information they have pieced together from other families in outpatient waiting rooms and hospital wards to try to make sense of their own family member's condition."

Schizophrenia draws the foremost attention of mental health services in China today (Boey 1997; Brassington 1995; Pearson 1996; Ran, et al. 2005). Pearson (1995b, p. 1164) notes that "Between 75–80% of psychiatric hospital beds in China are occupied by people diagnosed as suffering from schizophrenia." In 1997, the prevalence of schizophrenia in China was put at 6.55 per 1000 population, people with schizophrenia estimated to number 5.3 million in 1996 with 4.3 million living in rural areas (Ran et al. 2005). In contrast, the incidence of depression is deemed to be very low (Brassington 1995; Leff 1999; Pearson 1995b). As was the case in imperial times, depression is much more likely to be somatised in China than in the West (Kua, Chew & Ko 1993; Lin 1982). Kleinman (1986) paradoxically found in a 1980 mainland Chinese clinical study evaluating the efficacy of antidepressant medication for the treatment of patients presenting with a common somatised form of depression, 'neurasthenia' (神经衰弱),[2] that *fewer* patients labelled their illness as 'depression' *after* treatment than before, even though all patients had been informed of their diagnosis of depression pre-treatment and antidepressant medication had provided clinical improvement in eighty-seven percent of patients. This somatisation and denial of depression in China reflects a broader stigma against mental illness that has strong roots in tradition, as discussed earlier (Kleinman 1986).

The somatisation of mental illness is viewed by Western-trained health professionals as "maladaptive" (Cheung 1995, p. 164). For those inculcated with a biomedical understanding of health and illness, there is greater credence given to a more direct aetiological relationship between underlying pathology and clinical signs. In such an understanding, when one suffers from some form of psychopathology the expectation is for the pathology, for example, neurotransmitter imbalance, to clinically manifest in directly related psychological signs, such as psychosis or depression. When the relationship between underlying pathology and clinical presentation is more oblique, with conventional psychological symptoms suppressed or obscured by somatisation, the immediate cause-and-effect logic and the attendant understanding of disease process inherent to biomedical science is challenged. Rather than referring to alternative conceptions of health and illness for answers, such as normative cultural explanatory models grounded in life experience, challenges to conventional professional wisdom as a matter of course are characterised as deficient and problematic.

Such characterisations only add to existing cultural stigma and see many Chinese seek alternative pathways to care for a wide range of mental illnesses. As Cheung (1995, p. 165) has found:

> Chinese psychiatric patients travel a detoured course before arriving at psychiatric consultation. Studies consistently reported that Chinese psychiatric patients go through a process of self-help or a social support network prior to seeking professional help … For emotional distress, the Chinese generally resort to self-control, psychological endurance, pragmatic coping, and communication with their families or close friends rather than seeking professional help. The most common coping strategies are passive and resigned attitudes of learning to live with one's problems … Help-seeking is usually propelled by the recognition of somatic concomitants whereupon patients approach the general practitioner.

2. Although this expression linguistically was imported from the West via Japanese, Kleinman (1986, p. 154) states that "the concept and, more importantly, the social function are ancient. The concept that weakness of vital essence causes disease is a core category in traditional Chinese medicine and can be traced back to the classical texts."

Once again, the need for effective community psychoeducation addressing appropriate pathways to care for people with a mental illness is demonstrated. Such information can rarely be found in the Chinese media where mental health issues are "rarely acknowledged" (O'Donnell 2002, p. 8) and people with a mental illness "have a low or invisible profile" (Ran, et al. 2005, p. 129). Literary portrayals of mental illness abound, but, according to Brassington (1995), are rarely positive, for the most part emphasising the "alienation and hopelessness" (p. 205) of the illness experience and the unattractive physical appearance of mentally ill protagonists (p. 215). In fiction, mental illness once again is employed allegorically to symbolise broader social dysfunction, for example, the chaos and upheaval experienced during the Cultural Revolution. Alternatively, it reflects the stylistic features of a literary genre fashionable during the 1980s and 1990s in China, namely magic realism, where borders between the supernatural and reality are purposely blurred. Many leading contemporary authors address the issue of mental illness, including Can Xue, Han Shaogong, Wang Shuo, Zhang Jie and Zhang Xianliang (Brassington 1995, p. 201). The following excerpt is taken from Zhang Xianliang's (张贤亮) *Half of Man Is Woman* (男人的一半是女人), a controversial work published in 1985 in which psychotic hallucinations and delusions, amongst other post-traumatic disorders, afflict a protagonist suffering under the political and sexual repression of Maoist China (McDougall & Louie 1997):

> As I said these words, a great gust of wind came bearing down out of the branches. The willow and oleaster leaves were sent scattering, throwing dancing shadows on the ground. Out of the wind came a thick circle of inky mist, and out of the blackness came a tragic voice.
>
> 'It's all because the moon is not on course! It's come closer to the earth, and hence everyone has gone mad!' A dark face appeared, and then an ancient Venetian war-costume. Othello's eyes glared as he hovered above the ground. 'I have lost my courage too! Any coward could easily wrest my sword away from me. Evil has triumphed over good – does glory remain anywhere? Let everything return to oblivion!'
>
> He had been tormented in hell until he went insane, and his own conscience had played a part in his torture. His tragic voice was calling out a warning to every man who thought of killing his wife and then of killing himself.
>
> The black mist slowly dissolved, and the two spirits disappeared without a trace.
>
> Presently, the light of the moon brightened as the sky cleared up. My body felt as if it were riding along on my own line of vision, as I passed through the deep blue blue of the night sky, roaming through all the corners of space. From where I sat under the oleaster tree I could hold a conversation with any celestial

> body in the universe. Merely lifting my hand or my foot sent them out into the vastness of the world. I had thrown myself into the firmament.
>
> (Zhang 1988, pp. 168–69)

These literary representations to some extent reflect a continuing salience of supernatural understandings of mental illness amongst lay Chinese, in particular rural dwellers, despite the strong stance against superstition maintained by the communist government since 1949 (Phillips 1993; Ran, et al. 2005).[3] The government stance is echoed, for example, in state criticism of beliefs promoted by the Falun Gong movement at present. The currency of supernatural understandings of mental illness sees folk healing and shamanism, while officially unlawful in China, still commonplace (Kleinman 1986; Li & Phillips 1990; Ran, et al. 2005). In one study, Li and Phillips (1990) found that folk healers were consulted by at least seventy percent of people with a mental illness residing in rural China. The folk and shamanist practices used to treat mental illness, Li and Phillips (1990, p. 221) state, are syncretic, drawing on "aspects of Taoist, Buddhist, and animistic beliefs", with practitioners "explain[ing] illnesses in terms of spirits and ghosts, and … treat[ing] patients by intervening in the spirit world on their behalf." In the following, a typical folk healing experience encountered in rural Hubei province is recounted (Li & Phillips 1990, pp. 222–223):

> Mr. A was an 18-year-old peasant with 6 years of education who worked as a temporary laborer at a rural factory. Without any clear precipitant, over a period of 2–3 days he stopped eating, did not sleep, smashed household goods, stated that he was one of the 10 field marshals of China, and talked to himself, reciting the names of famous leaders and movie actors. After 3 days of this behavior his family members went to a local witch doctor and explained the problem. Without seeing Mr. A, the witch doctor told the family that an important deity was not protecting Mr. A from evil spirits. The witch doctor wrote the patient's name, date of birth, time of birth, and a request to the deity to take especial care of Mr. A on a large piece of yellow ceremonial paper. He then burned the paper, mixed the ashes in a bowl of water, and instructed family members to make Mr. A drink the mixture. This treatment, however, was not effective, so family members consulted another witch doctor.
>
> The second witch doctor came to Mr. A's home carrying a large sword and wearing a ceremonial hat and gown with multiple symbols woven into the fabric.

3. Pearson (1995b, p. 1166) has reported psychological explanations for mental illness from women clients in urban China, noting that "This is not a frame of reference that Chinese doctors usually share." She has also reported social explanations for mental illness by clients and families (Pearson 1995b).

> He burned ceremonial paper and incense and then sat down and chanted incomprehensible words. He then rapidly entered a trance state in which his voice changed, and he said that he was a spirit who had come to drive out the evil ghost. He picked up the sword, walked around the room several times chanting, and then entered Mr. A's room, commanding the evil spirit to go. Mr. A argued loudly with the witch doctor, pushed him out of the room, and refused to take the proffered ritual drink (noncompliance!).

State rejection of folk explanatory models of mental illness in contemporary China, at the same time, is complemented by promotion of the Western biomedical model and promulgation of the eugenic vision that characterised the republican government's utterings during the earlier modern period. In 1995, the Chinese National People's Congress passed the *The People's Republic of China's Maternal and Infant Health Care Law* (中华人民共和国母婴保健法), a piece of eugenics legislation which restricts the reproductive rights of people with a mental illness, amongst other disorders deemed 'undesirable' by the state (Dikötter 1998; Pearson 1995a). The law stipulates that "those 'deemed unsuitable for reproduction' should undergo sterilisation or abortion or be compelled to remain celibate … in order to prevent 'inferior births'" (Dikötter 1998, p. 1). It constitutes "simply a matter of quality control" of a burgeoning population from the Chinese viewpoint (Pearson 1995a, p. 1). Contemporary health manuals in China also see people with a mental illness, regardless of their state of recovery, as "unfit for reproduction" (Dikötter 1998, p. 137–138). Pearson (1992, 1995a), too, has documented the practice of sterilisation of people with schizophrenia in China.

Once again, a state-condoned eugenic vision that rejects corporal and psychological imperfection coincides with and so reinforces an aversion to mental illness (amongst other disorders) that attends Chinese patrilineal traditions. In present-day China, state-propagated biomedical conceptions that represent mental illness "as an organic lesion, a blot on the brain or a hereditary trait that is almost incurable" and consequently "advocate a strict ban on the reproduction of those deemed 'mad'" once again concur with traditional "folk notions [that] represent madness as a somatic defect running in family lines" (Dikötter 1998, p. 139).

In conjunction with the reproductive argument, the Chinese government also emphasises the importance of effective management of mental health issues to the maintenance of social order and stability, a key concern of the current regime. In April 2001, Chinese Vice-Premier Li Lanqing in an address for World Health Day stated that "mental well-being is an integral part of the overall health of people. To improve mental health is an issue related not only to the health of millions of people, but also to the social stability and security of human life and property of people" (Message of the Vice Premier 2001). Such statements, where people with a mental illness are "considered as a source of disruption and chaos, someone who is an inherent threat to public order and who needs to be controlled by outside forces", continue to be heard in government pronouncements concerning mental illness (Pearson 1996, p. 452).

Thus, in China, a state propagated eugenic vision and biomedical explanatory model of mental illness, together with the equating of mental illness with social disorder, potentially only serve to augment the already serious culture-bound stigma felt by Chinese individuals with a mental illness. As Dikötter (1998, p. 186) states:

> explanations, which might point to … the randomness of genetic mutations, are abandoned in favour of causal interpretations which often assign a clear responsibility to individuals. Individual agency has been overemphasised by medical determinism … [and] subordinated to the nation in the name of the collective health of future generations.

Stigma is also foregrounded in response to the demands of the market economy that now presides in China, particularly in competitive urban centres. Phillips et al. (2002), for example, have found that stigma experienced by Chinese families when a family member has schizophrenia is particularly evident in urban settings; amongst the educated; when 'positive' symptoms (e.g. hallucinations and delusions) are marked; and with persistent forms of illness. Stigma is also felt more profoundly by men and younger people with a mental illness (Phillips et al. 2002). This is because of the poor employment and marriage prospects that entail and the affect that these have on a family's livelihood in settings where traditional social safety-nets are rapidly disappearing (Fan & Karnilowicz 2000). In contemporary China, people with a mental illness, therefore, can readily be seen as unproductive and a burden – 'disembodied' – unable to contribute to the financial well-being of their family and carry out culturally prescribed social roles and expectations (Pearson 1995c; Traphagan 2000, 2004; Wong 2000).

Taiwan

Unlike mainland China, post-1949 the Chinese community of Taiwan was not subject to a radically new vision of the world which negated 'feudal' traditions and superstitions and upheld materialist and scientific understandings of phenomena. China's Confucian heritage continued to be revered by the Taiwanese government, in distinction to its rival on the mainland. For the lay population, traditional understandings of mental illness as sustained in republican China prevail, with a pluralist conception of mental illness commonplace in present-day Taiwan. This conception variably draws on ancestral and spiritual reckonings, family member transgression and heredity to explain mental illness (Kuo & Kavanagh 1994; Yang, et al. 1999), as well as "sorcery, hot/cold imbalance", "geomancy", "imbalances of yin/yang, bad fate" and "psychological and social stress" (Kleinman 1980, pp. 95–96). Kleinman (1980) claims that Taiwanese families simply opt for those conceptions that are most compatible with their particular experience and circumstance. Given these understandings it is not surprising that folk healing and shamanism remain commonplace in Taiwan, even more so than on the mainland (Kuo & Kavanagh 1994). Cheung (1995, p. 166), for instance, has documented widely practiced treatments for schizophrenia in Taiwan including "the use of herbs, secret recipes, and massage; Chinese- and Western-style tonics and non-prescriptive drugs; and folk healing such as shamanism, physiognomy, geomancy, temple worship, and spirit-calling." As on the mainland, few lay Taiwanese subscribe to the Western biomedical model of mental illness (Kleinman 1980; Phillips 1993), while a closer correspondence between lay and TCM explanatory models sees TCM conceptions more readily accepted by lay Taiwanese (Kleinman 1980).

This diversity in the explanatory models held by Taiwanese families reflects the myriad of coexisting aetiological possibilities provided by the Taiwanese historical experience: a deep Chinese tradition untouched by divergent political ideology, Japanese colonisation during the first half of the twentieth century and a fervent pro-Western (United States) outlook in the latter half. The strong influence of modernisation and embracing of Western ideas by the younger more educated outward-looking Taiwanese population born after 1949, who currently seek a more independent, local identity, however, may see less faith placed in traditional folk conceptions and greater acceptance of the Western biomedical model in the future. This is likely to be replicated on the mainland as well.

Migrant Chinese settings

The third Chinese community of interest to this study are recent migrants to Western countries such as Australia. Although Australia itself has a long history of Chinese migration dating back to the early nineteenth century (Ramsay 2004b), it is Chinese-speaking 'recent' arrivals that the Australian psychoeducational literature under study seeks to reach. In Australia, these predominately constitute migrants from mainland China, Taiwan and the Hong Kong Special Administrative Region of the People's Republic of China, and this pattern is broadly replicated in other Chinese emigrant destinations in the West, such as Canada, New Zealand and the United States. The explanatory models of mental illness for these migrants would be expected to strongly correlate with those of their respective 'homelands' as described above (Kleinman 1980).

This is confirmed by Lin and Lin's (1981, pp. 388, 392) study of stigma toward mental illness across the Chinese diaspora, which found that:

> The shame the [Chinese] family feels about the presence of a mentally ill member in its midst is, as a rule, intense and pervasive. This feeling is rooted in cultural views of the etiology of the mental disorder ... The moral view, a commonly held etiology, emphasizes "misconduct" as a cause of mental illness; deviation from socially prescribed behavior especially in neglecting the respect due to ancestors. Mental illness is regarded as a punishment for violating Confucian norms governing interpersonal relations, especially filial piety ... [T]he psychological etiological view of mental illness causes the family to feel ashamed ... [because the] psychological difficulties of the individual that have presumably precipitated or caused the mental illness reflect the failure, in the minds of the family, of performing their duty in guiding or protecting the individual in order to avert such disaster. The religious etiology implicates the family as having had ancestors who committed some kind of misdeeds. According to the genetic theory, mental illness tarnishes the family name, making it difficult for its young people to marry, which of course brings extreme disgrace to all those connected with the family ... *It is in this fear of the family exposing its own shame to outsiders that the origin of the stigma attached to mental illness in Chinese society can be found.* [original emphasis]

Mirroring the contemporary experiences in China and Taiwan, the explanatory models of mental illness salient to migrant Chinese communities living in the West can be characterised as heterogenous, encompassing traditional ancestral, spiritual, mystical, somatic and genetic causes, alongside the biomedical model that dominates most 'host' societies (Kleinman & Kleinman 1995). Given the salience of these explanatory models amongst migrant Chinese, the potential for conflict with the prevailing understandings of the host community, in particular their health services, is considerable. Lin (1985, p. 387) has documented "far-reaching mental health implications" for migrant Chinese arising from "the resistance of the Chinese to insight-oriented psychotherapy and the dominance of intra-familial coping in response to mental illness … where resolution of conflicts is attempted, consciously or unconsciously, by extrapsychic rather than intrapsychic mechanisms." Kuo and Kavanagh (1994, p. 556) have recorded a much more convoluted pathway to mental health care for migrant Chinese with a serious mental illness, typically comprising

> a protracted period of interfamilial coping with even serious psychiatric illness; followed by recourse to friends, elders, and neighbors in the community,

> consultation with traditional specialists, religious healers, or general physicians; and finally treatment from Western specialists.

The effectiveness of community psychoeducational literature in responding to this potential clash of understandings is explored in the ensuing chapters of this volume.

Chinese cultural explanatory models and community psychoeducation

This chapter has revealed that, while frequently somatised in Chinese societies, mental illness in fact has been recognised in China dating back to early imperial times. It has revealed that vestiges of the cultural explanatory models of mental illness salient to imperial times continue to inform conceptions held by many across the contemporary Chinese diaspora. The chapter has reported the influence of Western ideas introduced during the twentieth century, such as the eugenic vision, on the intellectual and governing elites in China, as well as the influence of ideological differences that emerged post-1949 across the Taiwan Strait. The chapter argues that in recent times these differences have likely diminished, with a heterogeneity in lay explanatory models of mental illness distinguishing present-day China, Taiwan and their respective emigrant communities across the globe.

This heterogeneity manifests a plurality of understandings relating to the causes, pathogenesis, pathways to care and appropriate treatment of mental illness. This situation for the most part contrasts with that in the West, where the biomedical model of mental illness is more universally accepted across contemporary professional and lay populations alike. Here, health professionals constitute the primary response when mental illness is encountered. In indigenous Chinese settings (China and Taiwan), however, the biomedical model remains confined mostly to health professionals and the primary response to mental illness varies. This mismatch between explanatory models of mental illness held by health professionals and lay populations in indigenous Chinese societies and between those held by health professionals in the West and migrant Chinese communities there has implications for effective community psychoeducation in both settings. This is explored in subsequent chapters of this volume.

The chapter also has documented the causes for the intense stigma toward mental illness that permeates the Chinese global diaspora. Stigma in Chinese societies has clear cultural origins based for the most part in Confucian tenets, such as patrilineal continuity, familial duty and responsibility, and social order and harmony. These have been legitimated, for example, by the eugenic vision propagated in China during the twentieth century by republican and communist governments alike and by the emphasis of the present-day communist government on social stability. Stigma sees individuals and their families reluctant to acknowledge mental illness due to the attendant shame and loss of face incurred. This ultimately has untoward consequences for the person with a mental illness. It is these very attitudes and behaviours that the psychoeducational literature examined in the following chapters seeks to overcome.

CHAPTER 3

The discourse of health and medicine

The act of disseminating new understandings and meanings occasions a discourse in the lay sense of 'conversation' or 'exchange of ideas', here between public health body and target community, albeit conspicuously unidirectional in manner. A view is presented by speaker or writer,[1] generating an expanse of language that mediates a matrix of contextual features within which the expanse of language, or discourse, is produced. This context entails not only the physical environment of text production (typically a health department office in the case of psychoeducational literature) but also the salient worldviews, beliefs and ideologies that inform and constitute the organisation producing the text. Consideration of these latter contextual elements is of particular importance to this study in that they, realised in language, will impact on reader reaction to the intended message, be it negatively or positively. That is to say, the way a text 'speaks' to a reader will be underpinned by the way an issue is conceived of and 'spoken about' by the text writer and, as noted in Chapter 1, this may or may not be conducive to effective communication of the intended message.

Explication of how the salient beliefs and communicative norms of the presenter of a message are mediated in text, be it spoken or written, is the province of the field of discourse analysis. Such an approach, therefore, forms the basis of this study's analysis of community psychoeducational literature.

A discourse analytic approach

Discourse analysis is a disparate field embracing diverse theoretical paradigms and drawing on a vast range of methodological approaches, depending on the task at hand and the epistemological disposition of the researcher (Schiffrin 1994). Jørgensen and Phillips (2002, p. 1) note that "discourse analysis is not just one approach, but a series of interdisciplinary approaches that can be used to explore many different social domains in many different types of studies. And there is no clear consensus as to what discourses are or how to analyse them." This is

1. Here, the usage may encompass singular or plural forms of the nouns, 'speaker' and 'writer'.

not necessarily problematic, discourse analysis being a burgeoning field of study for over three decades, provided that a clear statement of theoretical approach and explanation of adopted definitions is presented from the outset. This is the purpose of this section.

The preceding discussion has already employed two related but slightly differing notions of discourse: discourse as 'conversation' or 'exchange of ideas', arguably the dominant lay understanding of the term, and discourse as 'expanse of language' or 'text', one of the prominent definitions employed by many discourse analysts. The connection between the two notions is reasonably clear, namely, language as tracts of words, speech or communication, forgoing, at least in the author's opinion, the need to make any immediate distinction when both usages were employed in tandem earlier on. However, other common notions of discourse that feature in discourse analytic research move away from language as the sole concern, placing more emphasis on deemed normative beliefs or ways of viewing the world that are both constituted by as well as reflected in language use. It needs to be made explicit, therefore, how the expression is defined and employed in subsequent chapters of this volume.

Discourse analysis is frequently defined as the study of language in use (function) or language organisation beyond the level of the sentence (structure) in order to differentiate it from the descriptive studies of abstract language, usually isolated sentences, that characterise formal linguistics (Schiffrin 1994; Scollon & Scollon 1995; van Dijk 1997; Wood & Kroger 2000). There may be variable emphasis on function or structure across discourse analytic studies. Schiffrin (1994, p. 360) notes that where the

> focus [is] on structure, our task is to identify and analyze units [of language] … discover regularities underlying combinations of units, and make principled decisions about whether or not particular arrangements are well formed (or whether they conform to, or violate, sequential expectations). If we focus on function, on the other hand, our task is to identify and analyze actions performed by people for certain purposes, interpret social, cultural, and personal meanings, and justify our interpretations of those meanings for the participants involved.

Regardless, a structural approach can ultimately deduce useful functional conclusions and a functional approach does not preclude the consideration of structure, for example, how "the types of functions analyzed in discourse are realized in ways that create structures" (Schiffrin 1994, p. 339). As will become evident in subsequent chapters, while this study is primarily motivated by functional concerns corresponding to the use of language for communicative intent and effect across diverse settings, these determinations are dependent to a large extent on discourse structural considerations.

As mentioned earlier in this chapter, the primary focus of attention in discourse analytic studies may not necessarily be directed toward narrow language concerns but toward the dominant belief structures, hegemonic ideologies or 'social orders' that are at once realised in and shaped by, amongst other things, language (Jaworski & Coupland 1999). Here, language use "is assumed to be interdependent with social life, such that its analysis necessarily intersects with meanings, activities, and systems outside of itself" (Schiffrin 1994, p. 31). As such, tracts of language (texts) provide a means by which dominant belief structures and hegemonic ideologies, mediating the social experience of, for example, gender, race, sexuality, family, criminality, science and health, can be explicated and critically examined. This is because, within texts, discourses delimit meanings (Lehtonen 2000). They

> produce their own representations of reality. For example, discourses control the way ideas can be linked: what can be seen as a cause of a consequence, and vice versa. Hence, a discourse within itself sets restrictions to what can be said about … any topic. (Lehtonen 2000, p. 43)

Fundamental to such a notion of discourse is this interrelationship between text and discourse, which accords linguistic commonalities to texts that share discursive influences. Lehtonen (2000, p. 42) writes:

> As people produce meanings in discourses, the result may be texts (speech, writing, sound and/or visual images) similar to each other in the way that they share the central assumptions of the discourse. In this sense, the concepts of 'a text' and 'a discourse' are complementary … If we want to focus our attention on a particular case of a speech, writing, TV programme or other equivalent textual phenomenon, we talk about 'texts'. Again, if we attempt to seek for more universal patterns and matters that link the texts to other texts and human practices, we talk about 'discourses'.
>
> The concept of 'a discourse' thus defined is in a critical relationship to the notion of language as communication.

This study of the communication by public health bodies of a preferred conception of mental illness embraces such a definition of text and discourse. Text constitutes the tract of language under investigation, here community psychoeducational literature. Discourse comprises "ways of representing aspects of the world – the processes, relations and structures of the material world, the 'mental world' of thoughts, feelings, beliefs and so forth, and the social world" (Fairclough 2003, p. 124). These ways of representing the world are both realised in and constituted by texts and, as such, bind thematically and functionally related texts together.

Text, discourse and society

The above characterisations of text and discourse usually imply that the dissemination of a belief system or way of representing the world is strategic in nature, "tied in to projects to change the world in particular directions" (Fairclough 2003, p. 124). The intention may be to maintain the way a society, or section of a society, views an issue, or to promote a new way of thinking or viewpoint. The developing consumerist discourse mediating higher education in the West provides one example. More sinister, the intention may be to maintain or establish disparities in power distribution between groups in a society, usually to benefit a privileged group. Gendered and racist discourses are familiar examples that sustain male and dominant culture privilege, respectively. These are themes common to 'critical' discourse analytic (CDA) studies, whose research agenda, as Jørgensen and Phillips (2002, p. 63) note, lie in explication of

> *both* the discursive practices which construct representations of the world, social subjects and social relations, including power relations, *and* the role that these discursive practices play in furthering the interests of particular social groups … [and] in the maintenance of the social world, including those social relations that involve unequal relations of power. [original emphasis]

While the focus of CDA research for the most part is directed toward countering established political ideologies and attendant social injustices, its basic methodological approach is pertinent to most discourse analytic endeavours. This entails:

- analysis of the linguistic structure (the level of the text)
- analysis of the discourses … which are articulated in the production and the consumption of the text (the level of discursive practice)
- considerations about whether the discursive practice reproduces or, instead, restructures the existing order of discourse and about what consequences this has for the broader social practice (the level of social practice)

(Jørgensen & Phillips 2002, p. 69)

Fairclough (cited in Jørgensen & Phillips 2002, p. 68) represents such an "analytic framework for empirical research on communication and society" in Figure 3.1 below.

Linguistic features explicated in the text under study allow determinations of the salient discourses at work, both realised in text during production and constituted through text during consumption, facilitating the drawing of conclusions in relation to wider social or cultural issues. In the context of this study, differences

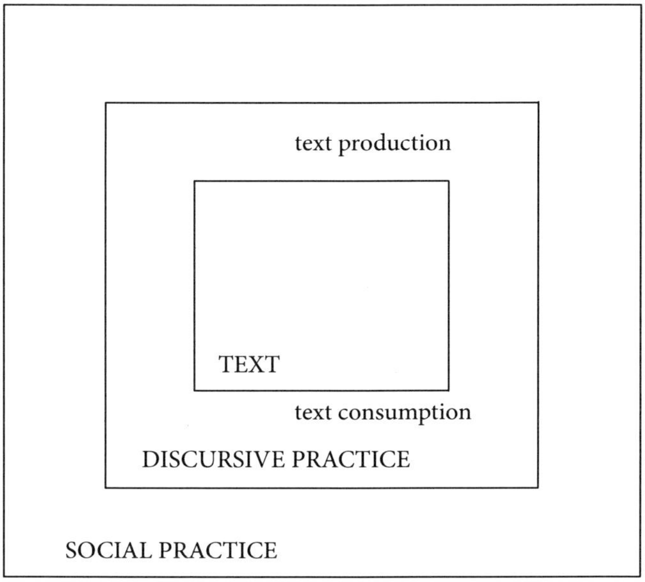

Figure 3.1 Fairclough's three-dimensional discourse analytic framework

in linguistic features apparent in Chinese language psychoeducational literature (text) drawn from across the Chinese diaspora allow determinations to be made as to the salient discourses at work (discursive practice). These are explored in relation to the broader communicative norms and salient sociocultural meanings attached to mental illness in Chinese societies (see Chapter 2, this volume) and their potential engagement, synergic or otherwise, with this discursive practice (social practice).

Discursive hybridity

The discursive practice or makeup of a text may draw on more than one discourse. Gendered and racial discourses, for example, can coincide in an instance of language use and serve to accentuate social distance or disempowerment (Fairclough 2003). In other instances discourses may be fundamentally antagonistic and compete for dominance (Fraser 1999). Representations of health and illness, for example, may draw on the biomedical conceptions that characterise professional medical practice or the more social understandings of everyday life experience.

Mishler (1984, p. 104) encapsulates these competing discourses as the "voice of medicine" and the "voice of the lifeworld", respectively. While antagonistic in reflecting distinctly different world views, one underpinned by science with the other by life experience, in any instance of health communication both voices may resonate to varying degrees. Coupland, Robinson and Coupland (1994, p. 90) state:

> The 'medical versus social' dichotomy is, in fact, difficult to establish as an absolute distinction in medical discourse, not least because *all* talk, indeed all utterances, articulate socio-relational meanings [original emphasis] … Even when a 'medical' frame apparently dominates in a specific medical encounter, participants will presumably pursue socio-relational goals in certain dimensions of their talk and these may be more visibly foregrounded at particular junctures.

Discursive hybridity, therefore, denotes a blending of discursive forms or 'voices' in an instance of language use, whereby competing voices differentially resonate with one achieving relative dominance, or synergic voices coincide with mutual amplification. Accordingly, the "forensic task of the discourse analysis", Jaworski and Coupland (1999, p. 9) state, entails "track[ing] how various forms of discourse, and their associated values and assumptions, are incorporated into a particular text, why and with what effects". This includes consideration of proportional and hierarchical dominance, given that "some discourses prevail and are more self-evident than others" while some "must struggle hard to be recognized at all as possible ways of speaking, let alone to reach the position of the dominant discourse" (Lehtonen 2000, p. 44). This needs to be reflected methodologically in the discourse analytic undertaking (see Chapter 4, this volume).

Mishler's aforementioned medicine-lifeworld dichotomy of representations of health and illness resonates in discussion of mental illness as well (Gwyn 2002). Harper (1996, p. 430) has stated that "professional accounts" of the paranoia associated with schizophrenia and related psychoses are ultimately "embedded in a deeper cultural reservoir of knowledge." Mehan (1999, p. 570) likewise observes that

> Two competing languages about the nature of mental illness have developed … One, called the "medical model", treats the issue in biological terms. Because the body is an organism, its various parts are subject to pathologies. Mental illness has developed as an extension of this way of thinking. The mind is treated by analogy to an organ of the body; it, like the heart, liver or pancreas, is subject to disease. As an organ, it can be treated in the same way as disease to other organs, i.e., by medicine, confinement, operations to remove diseased tissues. The cause and the cure of mental illness, like physical illness, is to be found in the biological realm … The second, called the "sociological" or "deviance" model, treats the issue of mental illness in social and contextual terms. Denying the analogy between the mind and organs of the body, mental illness is talked about in terms of actions and rules. Mental illness is the label attached to people who break a

> certain set of society's rules. Its origins are to be found, therefore, not in biological pathologies, but in the social context of relationships between people, people who identify rule breakers, people who apply labels and in extreme cases, institutionalize the rule breakers.

Recent research into medical communication, in fact, presents a more nuanced discursive distinction that distinguishes 'professional' and 'institutional' voices of medicine and recognises a 'client-centred' voice that draws together Mishler's voice of the lifeworld and latter-day concerns for consumer empowerment. A further complication emerges from the increasingly 'conversationalised' nature of communication in institutional settings, reflecting "the reproduction and transformation of different voices in new articulations" that inevitably attends discursive hybridity (Jørgensen & Phillips 2002, p. 151). Rather than subsume the voice of the lifeworld, institutional discourse can appropriate it in order to achieve its customary intent in a world increasingly unreceptive to bureaucratic practice (Sarangi & Slembrouck 1997). These discourses salient to medical communication and their potential interplay and intermixing are examined in the following sections of this chapter.

The professional voice of medicine

The practice of medicine has a long history and discrete traditions which have developed and cultivated within the health professions a distinct world view. Their way of representing the world is strongly grounded in scientific belief and protocol, and attaches great importance to materialist, rationalist and logical understandings of phenomena. Its fundamental tenets rely

> on the assumptions that reality can be rationally ordered by humans and that such an ordering, using the scientific method, allows people to predict and control much of life ... [T]his emphasis on science reflects the values of the rationalistic-individualistic tradition that is so deeply embedded in Western civilization (Samovar & Porter 2001, p. 63).

Fundamental to the scientific tradition is the belief that understandings of phenomena are substantiated and legitimated by means of rigorous testing regimes that are carefully designed to establish 'proof' or verify scientific 'truths'. These practices and truths for the most part "devalue emotion and intuition as sources of knowledge" (Macionis, quoted in Samovar & Porter 2001, p. 63) and "tend to prize rationality, objectivity, empirical evidence, and the scientific method" (Samovar & Porter 2001, p. 63). As has been noted earlier, in such an ethos the voice of life experience is significantly devalued, with "social, cultural, and biographical explanations" summarily dismissed (Dixon-Woods 2001, p. 1419).

Through their educational training and subsequent professional practice, health professionals acquire an expert knowledge encompassing "shared ways of knowing and seeing" (Roberts & Sarangi 1999, p. 480). These shared ways of understanding and representing the world find credibility and substantiation in the rigorous and well-established scholastic protocols of science, and this, in turn, is reflected in the professional's language of communication (Candlin 2001; Harper 1996; Mishler 1984; Sarangi & Roberts 1999; Selander, et al. 1997). Most obvious is the health professions' use of terminology that draws heavily on the language of science, producing, as Fleischman (2003, p. 473) observes, a distinct "occupational register … that gets passed from one generation of physicians to the next through the highly ritualized institutions of medical education." Here, differential utilisation of lexicon sees "patients' accounts [of illness] … set apart and relegated to the domain of the "subjective" – a negatively valued category in the world of science", with patient "observations … typically introduced using nonfactive predicators", such as ""state", "report", "claim", "complain of", "admit", or "deny"" (Fleischman 2003, p. 477). In contrast, Fleischman (2003, p. 477) notes that health professionals' accounts of illness are much more likely to be marked lexically by "factive predicators that put a stamp of truth/objectivity on the information that follows", such as ""note", "observe", or "find"". This register's reverence for professional opinion over patient experience extends even to the more "humanistic" fields of health care practice such as family medicine, where one finds "a sizable vocabulary for classifying and describing respiratory infections, but only one word for poverty" (Fleischman 2003, p. 474). This preference for the use of specialised vocabulary by health professionals, while providing for precision and specificity in communication and signifying professional collegiality and belonging, may also have unintended detrimental consequences for the health consumer (Wodak 1996). White (1995, pp. 113–115), for example, believes that in the practice of psychiatry such language may further 'pathologise' the consumer experience of mental illness and its attendant marginality:

> pathologising discourses are cloaked in an impressive language that establishes claims to an objective reality, [and] these discourses make it possible for mental health professionals to avoid facing the real effects of, or the consequences of, these ways of speaking about … those people who consult them[;] … ways of speaking … that reproduce the subject/object dualism that is so pervasive in the structuring of relations in our culture[;] … ways of speaking … [that] make it possible for mental health professionals to construct people as the objects of psychiatric knowledge, to contribute to a sense of identity which has "otherness"

> as its central feature. The success of these discourses is beyond question, and I believe that this achievement represents one of the truly great marginalisations of contemporary culture.

White (1995, p. 115) further argues that in the practice of psychiatry 'pathologising' discourses actually mask consideration of more experiential based, socially unpalatable explanatory models of mental illness:

> Pathologising discourses have the potential to bring to us a degree of comfort in a world in which it is becoming increasingly difficult to find this. The discourses make it possible to define those problems for which people seek help as aberrations. As such, they assist us to avoid the acknowledgment of the fact that these problems are very significantly of our culture, that these problems are products of our modes of life and of thought. The discourses of pathology make it possible for us to ignore the extent to which the problems for which people seek therapy are the outcome of certain practices of relationship and practices of the self … And the discourses of pathology make it possible for us to ignore the extent to which the problems for which people seek help are so often mired in the structures of inequality of our culture, including those pertaining to gender, race, ethnicity, class, economics, age, and so on.

It needs to be noted, nonetheless, that the utilisation of select or specialised vocabularies, subject to much attention in research on medical discourse, remains a phenomenon not unique to professional groups. As Valle (1998, p. 115) has observed, less conspicuous linguistic features of professional discourse remain of equal or greater concern:

> One of the most obvious social features of a professional community is that membership in it is based on training, often lasting for many years, usually taking place within the university or other comparable educational institution. In the course of this educational process, the novice or apprentice acquires an enormous body of knowledge, which is shared by the members of the community … [Their use of] specialized vocabulary is only the most visible sign of professional discourse; at least of equal interest is the *information structure* of the text, which reflects the structure of the professional community as a social and cultural entity. [original emphasis]

The discursive organisation and presentation of information in a text, therefore, will be symptomatic of the broader world view of the professional group that authored the text. In medical communication, this manifests in the pervasiveness of linguistic features that mediate the tenets characterising the professional practice of biomedicine, such as cause-effect reasoning, judicious practice and the elucidation of complexity (Gee 1999; MacDonald 2002; Selander, et al. 1997). Texts where these features dominate, therefore, are deemed to strongly resonate the professional voice of medicine. Chapters 4 and 5 of this volume make use of this relationship in explicating the discursive form of the psychoeducational literature under study.

The institutional voice

Medical communication not only mediates the expertise and shared world views held by health professionals but also the structured organisational environment within which the social practice of medicine takes place (Candlin 2001). The latter realises the institutional character of medical communication, whereby a pre-existing systemic order or organisational structure, or the agenda promoted by such entities, can shape, to varying degrees, the language utilised when health and illness is discussed both within the institutional setting and beyond.

Pelsmaekers and Geluykens (1995, p. 6) have stated that institutions and their attendant discourses are distinguished by their prescription of "roles" for organisational members and consumers, their specificity of "operation" and their delimiting of procedural "norms for … action." This institutional character is strongly contingent on the existence of a power differential exercised between organisation and consumer (hospital-patient), organisational representative and consumer (administrator-patient) or allied professional and consumer (doctor-patient), which ultimately privileges the former (Barton 2000; Fisher & Todd 1986a; Garcés 2005; Harris 2003; Iedema 2003; Mumby & Clair 1997; Pelsmaekers & Geluykens 1995; Sarangi & Slembrouck 1997; Thornborrow 2002; Wodak 1996). This power differential, as Agar (1985) notes in his seminal article examining (and entitled) institutional discourse, is sustained in order to effect control and, as a consequence, maintain the hegemonic position of the institution. This hegemonic position in turn allows "those in power the authority to pursue defined goals … to control resources and to act as gatekeepers, allowing options to some while denying them to others" (Fisher & Todd 1986a, p. ix–x). In the medical realm this is illustrated in the practice of health care bodies "using the institutional authority of their role [to] provide information in ways that function to persuade" which, while most likely well-intentioned, "denies patients the information they need to be active participants in their own health care" (Fisher & Todd 1986b, p. 23). More sinisterly, in the field of mental health, White (1995, p. 114–115) sees institutional countenance and propagation of a biomedical understanding of mental illness exploits what first and foremost is a professional conception of disease in order to "avoid accountability, and to retain and to extend on their monopoly on power." Such practice demonstrates a synergic interdiscursive juncture between institutional ('control') and professional ('expertise') discourses, an upshot of the hybrid nature of what is broadly known as medical discourse (Candlin 2001; Wodak 1996).

Control can be realised by institutional discourse in a variety of ways, including limiting or silencing the consumer voice, curbing or constraining consumer viewpoints and ways of understanding, exercising institutional imperatives or "directives" (what *should* be done), and managing the flow and presentation of information (Agar 1985, pp. 149–150). Institutions, not consumers, presume and define the posing of questions in an institutional encounter and, as such, largely control its direction. Institutions or their representatives determine what is significant (or noteworthy) and what is marginal (or unremarkable); what is permissible (or admissible) and what is precluded (or inadmissible). Institutions stipulate appropriate courses of action to which consumers are expected to comply. Consumers who fail to do so, whether through oversight, passive neglect or active choice, are usually considered by institutions to be uncooperative, problematic or insubordinate: the 'problem client' or 'troublemaker'. Institutions determine preferred positions or correct perspectives which are disseminated to consumer groups in order to effect belief change, with the consequence that individuals who fail to embrace the new institutionally-derived position or perspective are easily marked as intransigent or even, with the passage of time, deviant.

Through their membership of an organisation and their consequent acculturation into the established creed and normative system of arrangements and procedures that characterise the organisation, organisational representatives come to hold shared ways of knowing and seeing (discourses) that are reflected in the language of communication employed in the day-to-day operation of the organisation (Sarangi & Slembrouck 1996). Representatives of an organisation, therefore, are instilled with an "institutional culture" that mediates their behaviours in the workplace, including their linguistic behaviours in producing "texts whose purpose is, explicitly or implicitly, to regulate social behaviour" (Fraser 1999, p. 194). According to Iedema (1997, p. 73–74), these

> institutional discourses can be typified as concerned with the realization of constraint, or 'shouldness', on the one hand, and with the construal of levels of institutional enablement and power on the other. Realizing 'shouldness' according to prevailing institutional conventions makes possible hierarchical structures of power and authority, or the range of institutional positionings ... [It] creates institutional distance, which, by limiting the 'space for dialogue, disagreement, or differing points of view' ... tends to legitimize the Command involved.

Textually this produces a "linguistic subtlety and complexity [that] serves two purposes at once: the organization of human activity (shouldness) and institutional positioning (interpersonal distance)" (Iedema 1997, p. 95). Fraser (1999, p. 196) specifies these linguistic features of institutional text, noting that at the level of the sentence one characteristically finds a propensity for the use of "formal rather than everyday terms" and a "vocabulary … of defining conditions" often signalled by the imperative "must"; in sum, a "lexis" denoting "*regulation*" [original emphasis]. Sarangi (1998, p. 383) likewise considers the "overuse of nouns (rather than substituting pronouns)", "nominalization (verbs transformed into nouns)", "preference for passive structures", "use of noun strings (e.g., *healthcare maintenance organization*)", "parallel syntactic structures", "complex syntactic structures" and "[j]argon or special vocabulary (including abbreviations)" to be "distinct feature[s] of institutional discourse" [original emphasis].

Closer consideration, however, reveals that many of these sentential level features are common to professional discourse, as defined earlier. Another complicating factor in recent years is the aforementioned increasing 'conversationalisation' of institutional texts as part of a strategy to promote a more "consumer-friendly image" for organisations (Sarangi & Slembrouck 1996, p. 187). As a result, everyday language and communicative forms are becoming more commonplace in institutional texts. Sarangi and Slembrouck (1996) note that in many ways the use of "apparently non-coercive" (p. 144) plain language and the coopting of lifeworld discursive forms (e.g., narrative), "in which meaning becomes subordinated to instrumental effect" (p. 187), could merely constitute "further camouflage for introducing new forms of public control" (p. 9).

Consequently, as Valle (1998) called for earlier in relation to professional discourse, analysts of institutional discourse see value in shifting analytic attention to the presentation and organisation of information in texts (Sarangi 1998; Sarangi & Slembrouck 1996; Wodak 1996). Sarangi (1998, p. 384), for example, has noted that "[b]eyond the threshold of linguistic and stylistic features … information exchange in institutional settings is characterized by an asymmetry which is realized through interactional dominance." He states that in markedly institutional forms of 'talk', such as courtroom cross-examinations, asymmetry in information exchange is demonstrated by a distribution of turn-taking sequences in which "[q]uestions are formulated in order to constrain and influence what the witness can or cannot say in reply" (Sarangi 1998, p. 384). Thus, an important discursive feature of institutional talk (text) is control and the delimitation of boundaries, while in professional talk (text) it is professional rigour and conduct, that is, systematic, meticulous and scrupulous adherence to principles and practices laid out within a body of knowledge such as biomedical science (Candlin 2001; Garcés 2005). For example, the primary concern in the doctor-patient consultation is to ask questions "in a procedural manner to seek information from patients in order to arrive at a diagnosis" (Sarangi 1998, p. 384). While an element of control also exists, underscoring the hybrid nature of medical discourse, it is not of foremost concern, unlike the courtroom cross-examination experience.

Along with control, it can be seen that the crafting and maintenance of procedural rules and systemic boundaries distinguishes the institutional voice from the professional. Sarangi and Roberts (1999, p. 14) note that

> The notion of a profession stems from the idea of a vocation in which professed knowledge is used … An *institution*, by contrast, does not have the same roots in people as active agents. Rather it is an orderly arrangement of things which involves regulations, efficient systems and very different kinds of knowledge from that of the professional … It seems then that professionals, although most of them are institutional representatives as well, are endowed with a sense of agency based on knowledge and freedom … By contrast, institutional representatives in a bureaucratic organisation tend to underline objectivity and rule/procedure orientation of systems. [original emphasis]

Professionals, while frequently located in institutions and, on occasions, called upon to represent the institution, just as often, like consumers, have to negotiate institutional practices and boundaries. Institutional discourse, ostensibly, may appear to "share conventions" with professional discourse, for example, the practice of classification and categorisation, however, while knowledge-based rigour underpins the latter "[i]t is the combination of accounting practices and abstract rules which produce the shift from professional to institutional discourse" (Sarangi & Roberts 1999, p. 17).

In sum, this study sees language use in institutional text affirming and mediating institutional control and authority, and the rules and boundaries that sustain the control and authority. In the medical realm, this obliges (and subordinates) consumers (patients) to abide by medically-instituted agenda in order to obtain sought-after benefits (health care). Discursive imbalances and restrictions in the structuring of information presented in institutionally derived texts, such as those which inform consumers about illness and access to health care, will realise the power differentials and procedural boundaries that ultimately maintain the hegemonic position of the medical institution, here public health bodies. This phenomenon is explored in relation to the literature under study in the ensuing chapters of this volume.

The client-centred voice

A growing reconsideration by many of the dominant biomedical explanatory model of health and illness and the institutional practice of medicine has led to the steady encroachment, in recent decades, of alternative conceptions and representations of health, illness and the practice of health care that place greater emphasis on life experience and consumer empowerment. This movement reflects "a recognition of the poor quality of the evidence for many medical interventions, and of the existence of alternative, competing and contested views that may draw on lay ideas" (Dixon-Woods 2001, p. 1424). Alongside the aforementioned professional and institutional voices of medicine, this discursive orientation toward consumer interests and lay understandings, the 'client-centred' voice, has emerged as a consideration in contemporary medical communication.

Strictly speaking, the client-centred voice constitutes a 'counter-discourse' in that it mediates an alternative response to more established understandings of health, illness and the practice of health care. As mentioned earlier in this chapter, one distinguishing facet of this counter-discourse is its prioritising of life experience through "an increased emphasis on the patient's social context and experiences rather than solely relying on signs, symptoms, and demonstrable pathologies" (Dixon-Woods 2001, p. 1418). This responds to the emphasis traditionally found in medical communication on a narrow concern for "bodies" rather than "human beings and their perception of their real-world" (Selander et al. 1997, p. 188). The prioritising of the lifeworld over biomedicine is particularly cogent when considering mental illness, given that in the social realm the distinction between behaviour and psychopathology is often blurred (see Chapter 2, this volume); and that despite considerable pharmacotherapeutic advances in the treatment of mental illness in recent years the promise of universal, straightforward clinical recovery to date remains elusive.

There are sound communicative reasons for accentuating the voice of the lifeworld in medical communication. Bhui and Bhugra (2002, p. 6) note that acknowledging "patients' rich view of the world and of their illness within that world" through their expression of "social rituals, symbols in communication, forms of knowledge and illness narratives" leads to "a better understanding of their illness, including its meaning to them and their expected recovery process." Similarly, Selander et al. (1997, p. 188) have found in relation to dietary health educational literature that:

> If we really want to reach individuals, the information must be brought in line with individual knowledge, interest and ways of organizing knowledge. The opportunity for individual practice and experience should be provided ... If a patient receives information he/she regards as irrelevant for his/her needs or inconsistent with information from other sources, he/she is likely to refute the message due to lack of coherence, and the voice of medicine loses credibility. This means that information material should be directed from 'the voice of medicine' to 'the voice of the life-world'.

The lifeworld voice, therefore, is seen to achieve a higher degree of resonance with the health consumer by bringing the intended message closer to the consumer's frame of day-to-day experience. Dixon-Woods (2001) claims that the greater communicative efficacy that results from this legitimisation of the lifeworld experience leads to improved therapeutic compliance by the health consumer, providing benefit to consumer and health professional alike.

In addition to foregrounding life experience, client-centred discourse empowers the health consumer. Indeed, foregrounding life experience itself, for example, through the use of personal narrative, to some extent empowers the health consumer by contesting the intrinsic "social distance between patient and physician" and by allowing the health consumer "to assert a self … suppressed in the institutional discourse" (Ainsworth-Vaughn 2003, p. 460). This restores "the "personhood" of patients, who have been banished from a discursive stage on which organ systems essentially play out their dramas" (Fleischman 2003, p. 479). More distinctly, consumer empowerment promotes active choice, advocacy and involvement in therapeutic decision-making (Coulter, Entwistle & Gilbert 1998). Here, the health consumer is privileged as being capable, resourceful and adequately equipped to make rational choices and decisions, thus rejecting the prevailing professional perception of "patients as passive, there to be manipulated, and amenable to the objectives of the biomedical model were they not so incompetent" (Dixon-Woods 2001, p. 1425). In sum, empowerment privileges patient "autonomy" over professional "paternalism" (MacDonald 1998, p. 102).

Harper (1995, 1996) has examined the resonance of the client-centred voice in the mental health care setting. In one study he explores its operation in the context of auditory hallucinations that accompany psychosis, proposing alternative readings of the phenomena that challenge dominant biomedical explanations:

> For those seen as mad in the West the dominant narratives of madness revolve around psychiatry and the 'psy complex'. Many users of mental health services find the subject positions and identities provided for them in such discourses to be disempowering … '[H]earing voices' … need not imply pathology (many spiritualists, for example, derive great meaning from such experiences) … [E]xplanations need to include alternative perspectives from traditional psychological or psychiatric ones. Such an approach is useful in that users are given more of a choice in how to understand their experiences.
>
> (Harper 1995, pp. 352, 354)

Harper believes that due consideration of lifeworld explanations and commitment to choice are necessary conditions for a proper and empowering response to auditory hallucinations. In a subsequent paper, Harper (1996, p. 431) likewise reconsiders psychotic paranoia, noting that the paranoid experience can more usefully be seen as part of

> a whole tradition of 'suspicious interpretation' ... where meaning is derived from an inherent distrust of what is apparent and an urge to see what is the 'deeper' meaning. Suspicion is ubiquitous in everyday life. Although commonly denied, it helps us to understand the actions of others by speculating on intentions or motives. Such suspicious accounts are common in forms of gossip ... A broader viewpoint sees a conspiratorial or paranoid discourse as one used not only by supposedly pathological individuals but by all members of society.

Harper (1996, p. 432) goes on to argue the "meaningfulness" of psychotic delusions, given that

> the content of 'delusional' beliefs make sense when viewed from a stance informed by the believer's biography ... [and] that abnormal beliefs may have powerful functions for individuals, including: the maintenance of self-esteem[;] ... the conferring of special status; provision of comfort; provision of guidance; and removal of responsibility for negatively judged behaviour. Indeed, even a superficial look at the content of so-called 'paranoid' subjects in psychological research demonstrates the cultural embeddedness of these beliefs.

Harper (1996, p. 436) ultimately concludes that "there exists a wide variety of valid explanations – medical and other – for such experiences." His work on mental illness usefully brings to light the essential characteristics of a consumer focussed or client-centred discourse as it relates to mental illness and mental health care, namely: emphasis on the lifeworld experience with normalisation of difference and sanctioning of social and cultural interpretations of the clinical manifestations of mental illness; facilitating empowerment, self determination of subjectivity and resistance to psychiatric objectification; and the active provision of choice with open acknowledgment of multiple, diverse, co-existing explanatory models of mental illness. Such a definition is employed in the analysis of Chinese-language psychoeducational literature undertaken in the ensuing chapters of this volume.

A discourse analysis of Chinese-language psychoeducational literature

The chapter has laid out the discourse analytic concepts and broad approach adopted by this study. Discourse is viewed as ways of representing the world that are both realised in and constituted by texts. Texts are viewed as tracts of language in use. In mediating and constituting discourses, texts ultimately intersect with social phenomena. This study explores how the discursive form of Chinese-language psychoeducational literature sourced from across the global Chinese diaspora intersects with prevailing professional and cultural conceptions of mental illness.

The chapter has shown that the discursive character of medical communication is plural and hybrid, mirroring the discursive experience for most social phenomena. Here, discursive hybridity manifests in the differential resonance of discursive 'voices' deemed salient to the act of health communication, namely, the professional, institutional and client-centred. The professional voice mediates expert knowledge and specialised practice; the institutional voice mediates control and the setting of rules and boundaries; and the client-centred voice mediates life experience (Mishler's voice of the lifeworld) and active empowerment. The ensuing chapters will explicate the extent to which and the manner in which these discursive voices differentially resonate and blend within the public health literature under study. Jørgensen and Phillips (2002, p. 151) state that in "multivocal" texts such as those under study, the essential questions requiring answers are:

1. What characterises the different voices of the text?
2. When does each voice speak?
3. What meanings do the different voices contribute to producing?

The discourse analysis undertaken in this study will address all three questions by, firstly, elucidating what linguistic features actually mediate a particular discursive voice; secondly, explicating how discursive voices differentially resonate within a text both proportionally and hierarchically; and, thirdly, evaluating what underlying conceptual understandings of mental illness and normative communicative practices are represented by the blend of discursive voices realised in a text and how they potentially intersect with prevailing cultural explanatory models of mental illness. These questions underpin Chapters 4 and 5 of this volume.

CHAPTER 4

A discourse analysis of Chinese-language psychoeducational literature

Drawing on a notion of discourse and its hybrid realisation in texts dealing with health-related themes, as discussed in the previous chapter, this chapter explicates the discursive form of Chinese language psychoeducational literature sourced from three settings: mainland China, Taiwan and Australia. The extent to which and the manner by which professional, institutional and client-centred discourses are constituted in the texts under study are specifically evaluated. Attendant differences in discursive form presenting across the diasporic sites under study are also explicated. From an academic perspective it is interesting to examine how messages are communicated across different cultural (and diasporic) sites of action and contemplate the reasons for any existing differences. More practically, such analysis allows for judgements to be made as to the appropriateness of the form of a message communicated to a community, be it in indigenous or migrant contexts.

As discussed in the previous chapter, discourse analysis is a disparate field offering a wide choice of theoretical and methodological approaches to draw on for an analytic undertaking. Such diversity can be seen as fundamentally problematic to researchers from more conventional disciplines in that the soundness of study findings and their comparability with other studies are brought into question. However, work by leading discourse scholars such as Mann and Thompson (1992) and van Dijk (1997), in particular, have shown that once a theoretical approach has been clearly explained and soundly justified in relation to the task at hand, as conducted in the previous chapter, the range of methodological frameworks offered by the various disciplines that comprise the field of discourse analysis does not necessarily lead to conflicting interpretations of texts. On the contrary, the inherent diversity allows for a richness of textual analysis brought about by the opportunity to draw on a most appropriate framework or elements of differing frameworks in order to explicate the discursive features of interest to the researcher (Tannen 1990).

In the following section the discourse analytic framework employed in this study is presented. In so doing, its particular value to the analytic task at hand is clarified, namely explication of the discursive form of the psychoeducational literature under study in order to allow comparative analysis of site specific discursive features.

Rhetorical Structure Theory

Rhetorical Structure Theory (RST) views texts as comprised of networks of functional (rhetorical) relations that provide for textual coherence, at both local and global levels, and, at the same time, manifest the functional composition and discursive intent of a text. In this approach, developed by researchers William C. Mann and Sandra A. Thompson in the 1980s, rhetorical relations are seen to define both the relationships existing between a text's most basic structural units (clause or sentence) as well as those existing between larger text segments (groups of clauses or sentences). RST methodology, therefore, allows for the comprehensive description of the rhetorical form of a text at all levels of a text's organisational structure, "rather than selective commentary" (Mann & Thompson 1988, p. 243). As such, it is able to transcend alternative content-based approaches to discourse analysis that largely confine themselves to quantitative subject-matter-based determinations of text form and function without adequate consideration of organisational hierarchy.

The RST framework is a proven analytical tool of broad application, having been tested on a wide range of text genre, topics and length (Mann & Matthiessen 1991; Sanders, Spooren & Noordman 1992; Taboada & Mann 2006). In earlier work, the author successfully applied the framework in explicating differences in the discursive form of mainland Chinese and Australian news text (see Ramsay 1997, 2000, 2001a, 2001b). The current genre under study, community psycho-educational literature, likewise lends itself to RST analysis.

The starting point of an RST analysis is segmenting the text under study into constituent units. These units can be determined by the analyst based on convenience and relevance to the task at hand, but generally comprise "clauses, except that clausal subjects and complements and restrictive relative clauses are considered as parts of their host clause units rather than as separate units" (Mann & Thompson 1988, p. 248). In practice, this means that the vast majority of RST units constitute adverbial clauses and sentences; ultimately, consistency in analyst judgement is what is most required. Once the constituent units have been delineated (the numbers of RST units comprising texts in this study range from the mid-20s up to the high 400s, most being in the 100–200 range), the analyst needs to determine what form of rhetorical relation exists between units and groups of units (spans) comprising the text. It is important to note that determinations as to what relations exist between constituent units or spans are based on judgments of intended functions and meanings, regardless of "whether or not they are grammatically or lexically signalled", for example, by adverbial conjunctions or discourse markers such as 'therefore', 'although', 'however' or 'in order to' (Mann & Thompson 1988, p. 244). This is a fundamental principle of RST, as an approach focussed on function rather than morphology, whereby:

> a text is understood to cohere in the ways that it does largely by virtue of its relational structure rather than by virtue of overt markers signalling relations among its parts. In other words, connectives are better thought of as guiding the interpretation of a text than as necessary [or specific] signals of relations.
> (Mann, Matthiessen & Thompson 1992, p. 64)

By explicating intended functions and meanings, in linguistic terms the framework is "*pre-realizational, since it makes statements about how such meanings and intentions are structured and combined, but not about how they are realised*" (Mann & Matthiessen 1991, p. 233) [original emphasis].

While theoretically the set of relations that are deemed to exist between constituent text units or spans is potentially unlimited, in practice the number employed to analyse a corpus of texts is usually small: twenty-three were employed in this study (see Figure 4.1).

Rhetorical relation	**Abbrev.**	**Edited examples translated from psychoeducational texts**
antithesis	ant	Because schizophrenia can make people behave oddly and make them hear or see things that no one else can, some people think they are "possessed" by bad spirits. This isn't true of course. «ant« These are just symptoms of the illness which can usually be controlled by medication just like any other disease.
background	bgd	This is why it's so important for all of us to know the facts about diseases like schizophrenia so we can be more understanding towards people with the illness. »bgd» Because schizophrenia can make people behave oddly and make them hear or see things that no one else can, some people think they are "possessed" by bad spirits.
circumstance	cir	Just when she needs their help and understanding most, «cir« they say she's crazy and they avoid spending time with her.
concession	ccn	Although the problem affects between one to three percent of people of all ages, «ccn« it often begins in the teens and early 20s and is partly caused by an imbalance of chemicals in the brain.
conclusion	ccl	But it's hard for Kate's teenage friends to understand this. Just when she needs their help and understanding most, they say she's crazy and they avoid spending time with her. This means that Kate has to cope with, not just a frightening and bewildering illness, but

		also the loss of her friends. »ccl» This is why it's so important for all of us to know the facts about diseases like schizophrenia.
condition	cdn	Knowing more about schizophrenia also makes it easier for families to recognise the symptoms »cdn» if a relative develops the disease.
contrast	cnt	With normal adolescence, things like moodiness and depression only last for a few days at a time, «cnt» while with schizophrenia, the moods go on and on.
elaboration	elb	Kate is one of many thousands of young people in Australia with a serious mental illness called schizophrenia. »elb» It often begins in the teens and early 20s and is partly caused by an imbalance of chemicals in the brain.
enablement	enb	Anyone who is concerned that a family member may have signs of schizophrenia should contact their doctor, the Mental Health Team at their Local Community Health Centre, or: Transcultural Mental Health Centre »enb» Cumberland Hospital 5 Fleet Street North Parramatta NSW 2151 Tel: 840 3800 or 1800 648 911 for callers outside Sydney.
evaluation	evl	Some people think they are "possessed" by bad spirits. »evl» This isn't true of course.
evidence	evd	These are just symptoms of the illness which can usually be controlled by medication just like any other disease. »evd» In Kate's case for example, her doctors hope that medication will soon improve her condition.
joint	jt	One reason is that she often feels very frightened because she hears voices telling her she will be captured and locked in a cage. «jt» Another reason is that her behaviour makes many of her teenage friends feel uncomfortable.
justification	jus	People that claim that marriage can lead to an improvement in the mental state of a person with schizophrenia are utterly mistaken. »jus» There is absolutely no scientific basis to this claim.
list	lst	Conditions for referral: »lst» • illness stabilised, stable mental state and not posing a threat to others • suitable for open ward residency • possessing aptitude for work, motivation and capability to be trained • able to take care of personal hygiene • capable of undertaking vocational training and employment preparation • no infectious diseases

means	mns	Drama therapy is an adjunct therapy »mns» whereby therapists observe children's plays in order to gain insight into and treat problems.
motivation	mot	This is why it's so important for all of us to know the facts about diseases like schizophrenia. »mot» Knowing more about schizophrenia makes it easier for families to recognise the symptoms if a relative develops the disease.
purpose	pur	Drama therapy is an adjunct therapy whereby therapists observe children's plays »pur» in order to gain insight into and treat problems.
reason	rea	One reason is that she often feels very frightened »rea» because she hears voices telling her she will be captured and locked in a cage.
restatement	rtt	WHAT IS DEPRESSION? »rtt» What is depression? You first need to distinguish between feeling sad and suffering from depression.
result	res	It often begins in the teens and early 20s and is partly caused by an imbalance of chemicals in the brain. »res» Doctors think that this imbalance causes people with schizophrenia to hear and see things which aren't really there, and to have very disordered thoughts.
sequence	seq	Yonnie was rushed to hospital having suffered a cerebral embolism. »seq» Surgeons conducted an emergency operation. »seq» After the operation she remained paralysed down the left side of her body.
solution	sol	These are just symptoms of the illness. »sol» They can usually be controlled by medication.
summary	sum	... »sum» In short, when a person's mental illness reaches the chronic stage, their family on the one hand will need to offer even more care, patience, understanding and assistance, and on the other hand will need to cooperate with health services, and make appointments for clinics and attending rehabilitation sessions.

Figure 4.1 List of rhetorical relations employed in the study, with examples

In RST, the determination of what relations exist between text units or spans is based on reference to a set of relation definitions. These definitions clarify what constitutes a relation in question, that is, they provide the criteria by which an analyst can confidently and plausibly make a judgment as to what relation is in play in a certain instance (Taboada & Mann 2006). Systematic reference to relation definitions ensures analytic consistency and reliability, enabling validity to be achieved in a process that potentially remains open to criticism of subjective variation, given that relational judgments pertain to functional intent and are not primarily based on lexical or grammatical markers. Subjectivity is inherent to approaches like RST, as noted by Mann, Matthiessen and Thompson (1992, p. 52):

> To account for communication as one of the principal functions of language, a linguistic theory must be functional, in the sense that it must provide representations and draw conclusions about what the functions of particular uses of language are. If a linguistic theory of text structure is to be functional, judgments about the functions of texts and text parts must be made in the process of creating and testing the theory. In practice, such judgments are necessarily subjective, since they are made only by human beings who communicate, on the basis of what they know about their culture, their society, and their language ... We use this approach in RST because it is an effective way to develop functional descriptions of text, as a step toward ultimately coming to understand communication.

Two complete relation definitions are provided in Figure 4.2, illustrating how potentially similar relations, those of 'purpose' and 'motivation', can be distinguished

---

*Drama therapy is an adjunct therapy whereby therapists observe children's plays [N] »**pur**» in order to gain insight into and treat problems [S].*

Relation name:	PURPOSE
constraints on N [Nucleus]:	presents an activity
constraints on S [Satellite]:	presents a situation that is unrealised
constraints on the N + S combination:	S presents a situation to be realised through the activity in N
the effect:	R [Reader] recognises that the activity in N is initiated in order to realise S
locus of the effect:	N and S

*This is why it's so important for all of us to know the facts about diseases like schizophrenia [N]. »**mot**» Knowing more about schizophrenia makes it easier for families to recognise the symptoms if a relative develops the disease[S].*

Relation name:	MOTIVATION
constraints on N:	presents an action in which R is the actor, unrealised with respect to the context of N
constraints on S:	none
constraints on the N + S combination:	comprehending S increases R's desire to perform action presented in N
the effect:	R's desire to perform action presented in N is increased
locus of the effect:	N

(Based on Mann & Thompson 1988, pp. 274–76)

Figure 4.2 Relation definitions for the relations of 'purpose' and 'motivation'

analytically. For convenience, Figure 4.3 subsequently summarises only the 'effect' component of each relation definition.[2] The effect component, the most important of a definition, constitutes "a statement of some condition that is routinely achieved through the use of the relation" and, as such, "serves as a constraint against an inappropriate use of relations" (Mann & Thompson 1988, p. 258).

Rhetorical relation[1]	'Effect' component of relation definition
antithesis	R's positive regard for N increases on comprehension of S and the **incompatibility** existing between the situations presented in N and S
background	R's ability to comprehend N increases on comprehension of the **contextual information** presented in S
circumstance	R recognises that the situation presented in S **sets the framework**, usually temporal or spatial, for interpreting **N**
concession	R's positive regard for N increases on comprehension of S and the **ultimate compatibility** existing between the situations presented in N and S despite an acknowledged potential or apparent incompatibility
conclusion	R recognises that the situation presented in S can be **logically inferred** from information already presented
condition	R recognises that realisation of the situation presented in N is contingent on realisation of the **hypothetical, future or otherwise unrealised** situation presented in S
contrast	R recognises the comparability and the difference(s) yielded by the **balanced comparison** being made between the situations presented in two N or, on occasion, in N and S
elaboration	R recognises the situation presented in S as providing **additional details** about the situation or some element of the subject matter presented in N or inferentially accessible in N
enablement	R's comprehending S increases R's **potential ability to perform** the action presented in N
evaluation	R recognises that the situation presented in S **assesses** the situation presented in N and recognises the **value** it assigns
evidence	R's comprehending S as **credible** increases R's **belief** of N
joint	Equates to a rhetorical **conjunction**
justification	R comprehending S increases R's readiness to accept the writer's **right to present** N
list	R recognises that the items presented in multiple N are **serial parts** of a larger overarching structure

1. See Figure 4.1 for examples.

2. For complete relation definitions for the RST relations employed in this study, please refer to Mann & Thompson (1988), Mann, Matthiessen & Thompson (1992) and Fox (1987).

means	R recognises that the situation in N occurred or is likely to occur **by way of** circumstances presented in S
motivation	R's comprehending S increases R's **desire to perform** the action presented in N
purpose	R recognises that the activity in N is initiated with the **intention** of realising the situation presented in S
reason	R recognises S as a **cause** of N
restatement	R recognises S as a **restatement** of N where S and N are of comparable bulk
result	R recognises S as a **consequence** of N
sequence	R recognises the relationship of **temporal succession** existing between two or more N
solution	R recognises the situation presented in N as an **answer or solution** to the question or problem presented in S
summary	R recognises S as a **shorter restatement** of N where N comprises more than one unit

Based on definitions provided in Mann & Thompson (1988), Mann, Matthiessen & Thompson (1992) and Fox (1987).

Figure 4.3 'Effect' components of relation definitions utilised in the study

The RST analyst utilises the effect components of relation definitions in order to make the most *plausible* judgment as to the intended functional relation. As Mann, Matthiessen and Thompson (1992, p. 51) state:

> judgments about the writer or readers must be plausibility judgments rather than judgments of certainty. That is, every judgment of the completed analysis is of the form, *It is plausible to the analyst that* ...". In the case of the Effect field, for example, the analyst is judging whether it is plausible that the writer desires the specified effect on the reader. [original emphasis]

While it is granted that more than one relational effect seemingly may explain an occurrence in question, the analyst ultimately makes a determination based on what can most conceivably account for the writer's intention (Fries 1994).

Note that RST methodology recognises that some units or spans play a more central functional role in a text (nuclear) than others (satellite) (Taboada & Mann 2006). Relational asymmetry as an intrinsic element of text is substantiated by the research of the developers of RST, Mann and Thompson (1988, p. 266), as follows:

1. Often, one member of the [nucleus-satellite] pair is incomprehensibly independent of the other, a non-sequitur, but not vice versa. Without the nuclear claim, the evidence satellite is a non-sequitur, as is the background satellite without the nuclear span it illuminates.

2. Often, one member of the [nucleus-satellite] pair is more suitable for substitution than the other. An Evidence satellite can be replaced by entirely different evidence without much change to the apparent function of the text as a whole; replacement of a claim is much more drastic.
3. Often, one member of the [nucleus-satellite] pair is more essential to the writer's purpose than the other.

Mann and Thompson (1988, p. 271) conclude that, especially in relation to text whose primary communicative intent is persuasion, such as that under study, the nucleus-satellite distinction represents "an expressive resource that directs the reader to respond to the text in a particular and locally structured way. It seems to strongly influence the overall response that the writer intended." This nucleus-satellite distinction, along with the fact that RST takes into account relations between texts units and spans that may not necessarily be sequentially proximal, entail a hierarchy of governing relations within a text (Taboada & Mann 2006). This distinguishing feature of the RST framework is of particular appeal to the current study, as will become evident in the next section.

Sample analysis of psychoeducational texts

In this section, one of the psychoeducational texts from each regional corpus under study will be analysed in accordance with the above framework. This will serve as illustration of the analytic process for all the texts under study, given that length considerations do not permit analysis of the entire corpus to be presented in this volume. The sample text analysed from the Australian (AUS) corpus is 'Text 6'. The text comprises the content of a psychoeducational leaflet produced by the New South Wales (NSW) Department of Health's Multicultural Health Communication Service. The service provides public health literature in languages other than English to serve the local community. The sample text analysed from the People's Republic of China (PRC) corpus is 'Text 3G'. The text is one of many compiled in the edited psychoeducational monograph 精神疾病康复文集 (Selected Readings On Recovery From Mental Illness). The compiled texts had originally been published in a monthly psychoeducational newsletter 精神康复报 (Mental Illness Recovery News) put out by the 北京大学精神卫生研究所 (Mental Health Research Institute of Beijing University). The sample text analysed from the Taiwanese (TW) corpus is an extract of 'Text 6'. Given the length of the text only an extract can be presented here. TW Text 6 comprises the content of a psychoeducational brochure produced by the 財團法人董氏基金會 (John Tung Foundation), a public health charitable trust based in Taipei.

Identification details of the three sample texts are provided in Figure 4.4.

	AUS Text 6	PRC Text 3G	TW Text 6
Title	精神分裂症與年青人 (Schizophrenia and young people)	我的用药体会 (My experience of taking medication). In 精神疾病康复文集 (Selected Readings On Recovery From Mental Illness)	走出憂鬱迎向藍天 (Walk out of depression and into clear skies)
Author/Editor	NSW Health	姚贵忠主编 (Yao Guizhong Chief Editor)	財團法人董氏基金會 (John Tung Foundation)
Publication date	1996	2000	c2000

Figure 4.4 Identification details of sample texts

The initial steps in the RST analysis are demarcation of the constituent text units, followed by assigning of rhetorical relations. For each of the three sample texts these steps are represented in Figure 4.5, in both the original Chinese-language text and a literal English-language translation provided for reader convenience.[3]

(a) AUS Text 6:
精神分裂症與年青人 **1 »elb»**

清美與大多數十七歲的青年人不一樣，**2 »rea»** 她很少在空閒時間去見朋友們。**3 »rea»** 其中一個原因是她常常害怕，**4 »rea»** 因為她聽到一些聲音告訴她她將會被抓住和鎖在龍裏。**5 »res»** 有時這使她很不安，**6 »res»** 一致她不想去任何地方。**7 «jt» [w/ 4]** 另一個原因是她的行為使很多年青的朋友們感覺不安：**8 »rea»** 有時她好像是自言自語，或不是可笑的事，她也覺得可笑。**9 «jt»** 有時很難與她交談，**10 »rea»** 因為她會由一個話題跳到另一個話題。**11 »elb» [of 2–11]**

清美是澳洲很多千個患嚴重精神病 [名為“精神分裂症”(Schizophrenia)] 的年青人中的一個。**12 »elb» [13+14]** 雖然在所有年紀的人中，有百分之一至百分之三的人受這種問題的影響，**13 «ccn«** 這種病通常是在少年和二十出頭時開始。**14 »rea»** 部分原因是由於腦子內的化學品不平衡所致。**15 »res»** 醫生們認為這種不平衡導致患精神分裂症的人聽到和看到沒有真正存在的東西，而且他們的思想非常錯亂。**16 «cnt«**

但清美的少年朋友們很難瞭解這一點。**17 »evd» [18+19]** 正當她最需要他們的幫助和瞭解時，**18 «cir«** 他們卻說她是個瘋子，而且他們避免與她在一起。**19 »res»** 於是，清美不但要應付這種使人害怕和不知所措的疾病，她還失去她的朋友們。**20 »ccl» [fr. 17–20]**

---

3. The AUS Text 6 text's translation draws on, but is not identical to, the English-language version developed by the NSW Multicultural Health Communication Service. For demonstrative purposes, the English translation presented in this study is more literal to the Chinese version, which differs to a certain extent from the Multicultural Communication English version. This is not surprising given that, although the latter most likely would have been used as a template for the Chinese version, various negotiations would have been made in its redrafting into Chinese, taking into account linguistic and, hopefully, cultural differences. The PRC and TW texts were translated by the author with the assistance of Bai Ding.

因此，我們所有人都必須認識精神分裂症等疾病的真相，**21 »mot»** 以便增加我們對患該種病的人的瞭解。**22 »bgd» [23+24]** 由於精神分裂症可以使人們的行為變得怪異，並且使他們聽到或看到其他人沒有聽到或看到的東西，**23 «rea«** 有些人以為他們被邪靈"附體"。**24 »evl»** 當然這不是真的。**25 «ant« [23–25]** 這些只是該種疾病的徵候，**26 »sol»** 通常可以用藥物來控制，– **27 »cnt»** 正如其他疾病一樣。**28 »evd»** 例如，清美的醫生們希望藥物會不久改善她的症狀。**29 »mot» [for 21]**

增加對精神分裂症的認識並且會使家人們較易察覺該種病的徵候。**30 »res» [31+32]** 如果某親人患上這種病，**31 «cdn«** 就較易察覺到。**32 »evl» [of 30–32]** 這一點是重要的，**33 »rea» [34+35]** 因為如果及早察覺，**34 «cdn«** 病人就能更有效地獲得治療，**35 »res»** 他/她過正常的生活和不需要住醫院的可能性就較高。**36 »elb» [of 30–36]**

當精神分裂症在青春期開始時，**37 «cir«** 情緒的變化、個性的改變、抑鬱、難於集中精神、疏遠家人等警告信號有時會被誤解為少年人的正常行為。**38 «ccn« [37+38]** 如果是正常的青春期，**39 «cdn«** 情緒的變化和抑鬱等只會每次持續數天；**40 «cnt»** 但患精神分裂症的則會持續鬧情緒。**41 «jt» [w/ 39–41]** 正在患精神分裂症的少年與別人不同的另一點是他們有時會疏遠自己的家人和朋友們及停止自己的社交生活 – **42 «cnt» [43+44]** 而大多數少年則可能有時疏遠自己的家人，**43 «ccn«** 但通常不會疏遠自己的朋友們。**44 »sol» [to 37–44]**

任何人如果擔心自己的家人可能有精神分裂症的徵兆，**45 «cdn«** 就應該與醫生、當地的社區保健中心 (Community Health Centre) 的精神健康隊、或超越文化精神健康中心 (Transcultural Mental Health Centre) 聯絡，**46 »enb»** 地址: Cumberland Hospital, 5 Fleet Street, North Parramatta, NSW 2151, 電話: (02) 9840 3800。在雪梨都市以外的地方可以打 1800 648 911。**47 »mot» [for 45–47]** 該中心可以幫助人們與講他們的母語的精神保健專業人士聯絡。**48 «jt» [w/ 46]** 精神分裂症會 (Schizophrenia Fellowship) 也可以為精神分裂症病人和其家人提供資料和支援。**49 »enb»** 電話: (02) 9879 2600 **50**

Schizophrenia and Young People **1 »elb»**

Kate is unlike most 17 year-olds. **2 »rea»** She spends very little of her leisure time seeing friends. **3 »rea»** One reason is that she often feels very frightened, **4 »rea»** because she hears voices telling her she will be captured and locked in a cage. **5 »res»** Sometimes this makes her feel very anxious, **6 »res»** causing her not to want to go out anywhere. **7 «jt» [w/ 4]** Another reason is that her behaviour makes many of her teenage friends feel uncomfortable: **8 »rea»** Sometimes she seems to be talking to herself, or she laughs at things which aren't funny. **9 «jt»** Sometimes her conversation is difficult to follow, **10 »rea»** because she jumps from one topic to another. **11 »elb» [of 2–11]**

Kate is one of many thousands of young people in Australia with a serious mental illness called schizophrenia. **12 »elb» [13+14]** Although the problem affects between one to three percent of people of all ages, **13 «ccn«** it often begins in the teens and early 20s. **14 »rea»** It is partly caused by an imbalance of chemicals in the brain. **15 »res»** Doctors think that this imbalance causes people with schizophrenia to hear and see things which aren't really there, and to have very disordered thoughts. **16 «cnt«**

But it's hard for Kate's teenage friends to understand this. **17 »evd» [18+19]** Just when she needs their help and understanding most, **18 «cir«** they say she's crazy, and they avoid spending time with her. **19 »res»** This means that Kate has to cope with not just a frightening and bewildering illness, but also the loss of her friends. **20 »ccl» [fr. 17–20]**

Thus, all of us need to know the facts about diseases like schizophrenia, **21 »mot»** so we can be more understanding towards people with the illness. **22 »bgd» [23+24]** Because schizophrenia can make people behave oddly, and make them hear or see things that no one else can, **23 «rea«** some people think they are "possessed" by bad spirits. **24 »evl»** This isn't true of course. **25 «ant« [23–25]** These are just symptoms of the illness. **26 »sol»** They can usually be controlled by medication – **27 »cnt»** just like any other disease. **28 »evd»** In Kate's case, for example, her doctors hope that medication will soon improve her condition. **29 »mot» [for 21]**

Knowing more about schizophrenia also makes it easier for families to recognise the symptoms of this disease. **30 »res» [31+32]** If a relative develops the disease, **31 «cdn«** then it'll be easier to detect. **32 »evl» [of 30–32]** This is important, **33 »rea» [34+35]** because if it's detected early, **34 «cdn«** sufferers can receive more effective treatment, **35 »res»** giving them a better chance of leading a normal life and staying out of hospital. **36 »elb» [of 30–36]**

When schizophrenia begins in adolescence, **37 «cir«** the warning signs such as changing moods, personality changes, depression, difficulty concentrating and withdrawing from the family are sometimes assumed to be just normal teenager behaviour. **38 «ccn« [37+38]** If it were regular adolescence, **39 «cdn«** things like moodiness and depression would only last for a few days at a time; **40 «cnt»** but in the case of people with schizophrenia the moods go on and on. **41 «jt» [w/ 39–41]** Another point of difference in the case of teenagers who are developing schizophrenia is that they sometimes will withdraw from their family and friends as well as from their social life – **42 «cnt» [43+44]** but while most teenagers may withdraw from their families sometimes, **43 «ccn«** they usually do not withdraw from their friends. **44 »sol» [to 37–44]**

If anyone is concerned that a family member may have signs of schizophrenia, **45 «cdn«** they should contact their doctor, the mental health team at their local Community Health Centre, or the Transcultural Mental Health Centre, **46 »enb»** Address: Cumberland Hospital, 5 Fleet Street, North Parramatta, NSW 2151, Tel: (02) 9840 3800. Callers outside Sydney can phone 1800 648 911. **47 »mot» [for 45–47]** The centre can help put people in touch with mental health professionals who speak their language. **48 «jt» [w/ 46]** The Schizophrenia Fellowship can also provide information and support to people with schizophrenia and their families. **49 »enb»** Telephone: (02) 9879 2600. **50**

(b) PRC Text 3G:

我的用药体会 **1 »elb»**

我是1993年患精神分裂症的，**2 »elb» [3+4]** 当时总觉得周围的人跟踪自己，觉得公路上跑的汽车牌号都跟自己有关，**3 «jt»** 好像别人说话干事都是针对自己的，电视里的镜头也含沙射影地说自己。**4 »seq»** 这时，我按医嘱每天服用14片奋乃静，**5 »seq» [6–8]** 服用了近一个月，**6 «cir«** 幻觉和跟踪感就消失了。**7 «ccn« [6+7]** 但伴随的心慌、烦躁不安和孤独感仍然存在。**8 »seq» [9+10]** 后经继续服用奋乃静三个月，**9 «cir«** 我的身体恢复得和正常人没多大的区别了。**10 »seq» [11+12]**

因嗜睡影响工作，**11 «rea«** 我于1994年8月停药。12 **»seq»** 此后没多长时间，病就复发了，症状和以前差不多。**13 »seq»** 母亲发现后，马上让我服用奋乃静，**14 »seq» [15+16]** 过了一段时间，**15 «cir«** 又恢复了正常。**16 »seq»**

1996年，我结识了一个男朋友，**17 »seq»** 对方迫切要求结婚生小孩。**18 »seq» [19–21]** 我担心由于用药，**19 «rea«** 生育残疾儿，**20 »res»** 于1997年初又停药了。**21 »seq» [22+23]** 停药后病情再度复发，而且比以前还厉害，**22 »evd»** 不但有幻觉，而且还想死，想卧轨、跳楼。**23 »seq» [24+25]** 妈妈又领我到医院诊治，**[24] »res»** 医生让我服用维思通和百优解，**25 »seq» [26+27]** 服了近两个月，**26 «cir«** 效果不明显，而且月经也不正常了，**27 »seq» [28+29]** 后又改用奋乃静、佳静安定等药，**28 «cir«** 恢复了正常。**29 »seq»**

几年来我亲身体会到：**»lst»**

(1) 患精神分裂症必须坚持长期用药，**30 »ant»** 不能吃吃停停。**31**
(2) 用药要因人而异，**32 «rea«** 找到了适合自己的药 **33 «cir«** 就不要轻易换药。**34 »mot» [for 33+34]** 我的病第二次复发时，**35 «cir«** 看到电视上说维思通是最好的药，**36 «rea«** 就改用了维斯通，**37 »res»** 结果出现坐立不安、月经失调等副作用，**38 »elb» [39+40]** 不但原来的症状没去掉，**39 »cnt»** 反而添了其他症状。**40 »seq» [41+42]** 后来经医生调整，仍服用奋乃静和佳静安定，**41 «mns«** 很快恢复了正常。**42**
(3) 换药一定要遵医嘱，逐渐调整，**43 »ant»** 不能朝令夕改，急于求成。**44**

My Experience of Taking Medication **1 »elb»**

I developed schizophrenia in 1993. **2 »elb» [3+4]** At the time I always felt that people around me were following me, that the number plates on the cars running on the road had something to do with me. **3 «jt»** It seemed that the words and actions of other people were always aimed at me, that the scenes on television were maliciously talking about me. **4 »seq»** At the time every day I took 14 tablets of Perphenazine according to doctors' advice. **5 »seq» [6–8]** After I had taken this medication for nearly a month, **6 «cir«** the hallucinations and paranoia disappeared, **7 «ccn« [6+7]** but the anxiety, restlessness and feeling of loneliness that accompanied the illness still remained. **8 »seq» [9+10]** After having taken Perphenazine continuously for three months, **9 «cir«** my body recovered to a level not so different to normal people. **10 »seq» [11+12]**

Since tiredness affected my work, **11 «rea«** I stopped taking medication in August 1994. **12 »seq»** Not long thereafter my illness recurred with symptoms much as before. **13 »seq»** After finding this out my mother made me take Perphenazine straight away. **14 »seq» [15+16]** After a period of time, **15 «cir«** I again returned to normal. **16 »seq»**

In 1996 I met a boyfriend. **17 »seq»** He was keen to get married and have children. **18 »seq» [19–21]** Because I was taking medication **19 «rea«** I was afraid of giving birth to a disabled child **20 »res»** and in the beginning of 1997 I again stopped taking medication. **21 »seq» [22+23]** After that the illness reappeared once again and worse than before. **22 »evd»** Not only did I have hallucinations but I also wanted to die, to lie on the railway line or jump from an apartment building. **23 »seq» [24+25]** Again my mum took me to hospital to get diagnosed and treated, **[24] »res»** the doctors asking me to take Risperidone and Prozac. **25 »seq» [26+27]** After taking them for nearly two months **26 «cir«** the results were not obvious and my periods became irregular. **27 »seq» [28+29]** Then I changed to medications such as Perphenazine and Xanax **28 «cir«** and I returned to normal. **29 »seq»**

Over the years I have personally realized that: **»lst»**
(1) People with schizophrenia must persist in taking medication over the longer term; **30 »ant»** one cannot stop taking medication at will. **31**
(2) Medication will be different for different people. **32 «rea«** When you find medication that suits you **33 «cir«** do not change it rashly. **34 »mot» [for 33+34]** In my second relapse, **35 «cir«** having seen on television that Risperidone was the best medication, **36 «rea«** I switched to using Risperidone. **37 »res»** The result was that I developed side effects like restlessness and irregular periods. **38 »elb» [39+40]** Not only did the original symptoms not abate, **39 »cnt»** but on the contrary other symptoms emerged. **40 »seq» [41+42]** Later on, through adjustments by the doctor and taking Perphenazine and Xanax, **41 «mns«** I quickly returned to normal. **42**
(3) Only change medication on doctors' advice and do it gradually. **43 »ant»** Do not change at will, eager for immediate results. **44**

(c) TW Text 6 (extract):

走出憂鬱迎向藍天 **1 »elb»**

你最近是不是常常情緒低落鬱悶？**2 »sol» [3+4]** 如果你發現自己或身邊的親友情緒低落持續兩週以上，或者對各種活動嗜好或交朋友都失去了興趣，缺乏毅力鬥志，**3 «cdn«** 對於這樣早期發現憂鬱症的警訊更要注意。。。。。。**4 »elb» …**

»lst» 憂鬱症案例1 **146 »elb»** 生活上的小丑 **147 »elb»**

給別人歡樂的小丑，也不該忘記給自己歡笑 **148 »elb»**

「生活上的小丑」是她給自己的暱稱，**149 »elb»** 幫助他人、傾聽別人心中的聲音、帶給大家歡樂是她所以為的要務，**150 »elb» [151+152]** 她悄悄地告訴自己「我是別人訴苦、信任的對象，有問題時，我應該可以自己處理」，**151 »res»** 於是習慣了將難過往自己的肚裡吞。**152**

»elb» [of 148] [153+154] 因為她本身完美主義的性格，153 «rea« 常給自己很高的期許，154 »seq» [155–157] 在服務他人的同時，155 «cir« 因為個性急又求好，156 «rea« 以至於造成更大的壓力。157 »seq» [158+159] 漸漸地，在她帶給別人快樂的同時，158 «cir« 卻發現自己的身體愈來愈不對勁，拉肚子、嘔吐、無法睡覺、拿東西會顫抖等症狀一一出現。159 »seq» [160+161]

因為身邊的朋友曾有過憂鬱的現象，也常從閱讀報章雜誌上，知道一些憂鬱症的早期症狀，160 «rea« 她立即警覺到自己的異常。161 »seq» 她說「小丑也不該忘了給自己歡笑！」162 »seq» [163+164] 經過一陣子的不舒服之後，163 «cir« 馬上向精神科求助。164 »seq» [165+166] 剛開始無法接受醫生開的藥，165 »rea» 因為吃藥會讓她昏睡，166 »seq» [167–169] 即使是生病 167 «ccn« 心中仍掛念著：「我要趕快醫好，我要工作！」168 »res» 不僅要求住院治療，更大聲地對醫生說：「你再讓我這樣昏昏沉沉的，我就要自殺！」169 »seq» 憂鬱症在她的生理上造成很大的痛苦，170 »evd» 許多事不能再如自己的理想達成：「為什麼不快點好？ 為什麼要這樣過日子？」171 »evd» [of 170] 也開始出現暴食，要不然就沒辦法飲食的極端現象。172 »seq»

活潑的人還是會得到憂鬱症» 173 »elb»

在許多事與願違下，174 «cir« 唯一持續的是看醫生、聽從指示，也開始尋求各方面的生活協助：175 »elb» [176–183] »lst» 繼續參加爬山、唱歌、跳舞等休閒活動；176 閱讀書籍資料了解就醫吃藥的目的；177 學習與他人分享心中的感覺；178 降低對自己的要求，179 »mns» [180+181] 當很著急時，180 «cir« 提醒自己慢一點又有什麼關係；181 適時抒發壓抑的情緒；182 最重要的是勇敢地向周遭的朋友坦誠：「我有憂鬱症」。183 »seq»

她說：「活潑的人，還是會得憂鬱症的！」184 »elb» [185–193] 以前寧願自己一個人承受壓力，185 »ant» 不願被打擾，不願接受他人的好意，186 »res» 因此容易與人產生衝突。187 «cnt» 現在想開了，主動讓別人知道自己的情況與想法，188 »res» [189+190] 當別人了解時，189 «cir« 就會去配合；190 «cnt» 彼此不了解往往會產生心結與誤會，191 »res» 惡性循環的結果更可能導致病患無法獲得認同與支持反而更沮喪，192 »res» 影響病情的康復。193 »seq»

現在的她，繼續盡責地做著生活上的小丑，給予病友們同理心及適時的安慰，194 »res» 讓他們可以得到最直接且立即的協助。195 »elb» [of 194+195] 另一方面，她學會了如何紓解工作上的壓力，也知道如何去與關心她的人溝通並對自己妥協。196 »seq» [197+198] 小丑不再只是帶給他人歡笑，197 «ant« 自己也活得比以前快樂且充滿自信。198

»lst» 案例2 199 »elb» 青春夢碎 200 »elb» …

Walk out of Depression and into Clear Skies 1 »elb»

Have you often been feeling down or depressed lately? 2 »sol» [3+4] If you find that you or your family and friends around you have been continuously feeling down for more than two weeks, have lost interest in all kinds of activities, hobbies or making friends and are lacking in drive and willpower, 3 «cdn« you need to pay attention to these early warning signs of depression …… 4 »elb» …

»lst» Case 1 of Depression 146 »elb» Clown in Life 147 »elb»

The Clown Who Brings Joy to Other People Should Not Forget to Laugh Heartily for Oneself 148 »elb»

"Clown in life" is the nickname she gave herself. 149 »elb» Her key duty, she thought, was to help others, to listen attentively to their heartfelt voices and bring joy to everyone. 150 »elb» [151+152] She quietly told herself "I am the object of other people's grievances and trust. When there is a problem I ought to be able to deal with it myself." 151 »res» Thus, she became accustomed to internalising her sadness. 152

»elb» [of 148] [153+154] Because of her perfectionist temperament 153 «rea« she often set herself high expectations. 154 »seq» [155–157] While serving other people, 155 «cir« because of her impatient and exacting personality, 156 «rea« she placed even greater pressure on herself. 157 »seq» [158+159] Gradually, at the same time as bringing joy to other people, 158 «cir« she found her own health deteriorating more and more, with symptoms like diarrhoea, vomiting, insomnia and intention tremors appearing one after another. **159 »seq» [160+161]**

Because a friend of hers had once experienced depression and knowing a bit about the early signs of depression from reading newspapers and magazines, **160 «rea«** she immediately became aware of her abnormality. **161 »seq»** She said "the clown should not forget to laugh heartily for oneself!" **162 »seq» [163+164]** Following a period of time of feeling unwell, **163 «cir«** she immediately sought psychiatric help. **164 »seq» [165+166]** At the very beginning she was unable to tolerate the medication she was prescribed, **165 »rea»** because the medication would make her drowsy. **166 »seq» [167–169]** Even though ill, **167 «ccn«** in her heart she still thought "I want to quickly be cured. I want to work." **168 »res»** Not only did she demand to be treated in hospital but even more loudly said to the doctor "if you ever make me dizzy like this again I will kill myself!" **169 »seq»** Depression caused her tremendous physiological suffering. **170 »evd»** She could no longer achieve many things as she ideally wished to: "Why can't I get better faster? Why must I live like this?" **171 »evd» [of 170]** Extreme episodes of binge eating or loss of appetite also began to emerge. **172 »seq»**

Lively People Can Still Get Depression **173 »elb»**

With many things not turning out as planned, **174 «cir«** the only things she continued to do were seeing the doctor, following his or her advice and starting to seek out various life outlets: **175 »elb» [176–183] »lst»** continuing to take part in leisure activities such as mountain climbing, singing and dancing; **176** reading books and materials to find out the purpose of seeing the doctor and taking medication; **177** learning to share heartfelt feelings with others; **178** reducing demands on herself **179 »mns» [180+181]** by, when feeling anxious, **180 «cir«** reminding herself to slow down a bit and think what does it have to do with; **181** expressing repressed feelings at the right moment; **182** and, most importantly, being bravely candid and honest to friends around her: "I have depression." **183 »seq»**

She said "lively people can still get depression!" **184 »elb» [185–193]** Previously she would rather bear pressure alone, by herself. **185 »ant»** She was not willing to be disturbed and not willing to accept other people's kindness. **186 »res»** Consequently it was easy for conflict with people to arise. **187 «cnt»** Now she thinks to take the initiative and make other people aware of her own circumstances and ideas. **188 »res» [189+190]** When other people understand, **189 «cir«** they can fit in with her; **190 «cnt»** not understanding each other can often give rise to deep-rooted problems and misunderstandings. **191 »res»** The outcome of a vicious circle will more likely lead to the ill person being unable to gain acknowledgment and support and instead being more dispirited, **192 »res»** affecting recovery from the illness. **193 »seq»**

Nowadays, she continues to fulfil her duty to be the clown in life, giving fellow sufferers empathy and comfort at the right moment. **194 »res»** This allows them to be able to obtain the most direct and immediate assistance. **195 »elb» [of 194+195]** On the other hand she has learnt how to ease the pressure of work and knows how to communicate with people who care for her and how to make self-compromise. **196 »seq» [197+198]** The clown no longer merely brings laughter to others; **197 «ant«** she also lives more happily and brimming with more self-confidence than before. **198**

»lst» Case 2 **199 »elb»** Youthful Dream Shattered **200 »elb» …**

Figure 4.5 Demarcation of RST units comprising the sample texts and assignment of RST relations

The next analytic step entails constructing the RST diagram for the text in order to reveal its governing hierarchy of rhetorical relations. The schematic conventions employed by the author in earlier studies (Ramsay 1997, 2000, 2001a) are employed here due to their clarity in illustration of rhetorical hierarchy. These draw heavily on Fox's (1987) RST conventions. Figure 4.6 provides an example of a 'purpose' relational schema under this convention.

Drama therapy is an adjunct therapy whereby therapists observe children's plays ***1*** *»**pur**» in order to gain insight into and treat problems. 2*

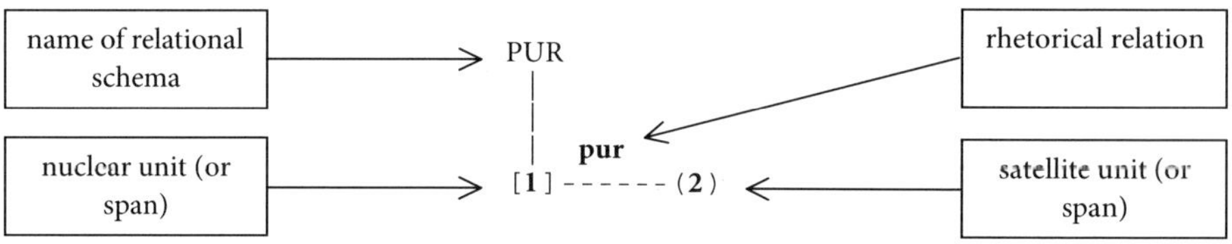

Figure 4.6. RST 'purpose' relational schema

Not surprisingly, the name of a schema typically matches the relation it depicts. The exception in this convention is the 'Issue' (ISS) schema, which encompasses the relations of elaboration, background and evidence. This is because elaboration, background or evidence satellites can concurrently originate from the one nuclear claim, known as the 'issue'. Such a situation does not eventuate with other relations' schematic representations.

Hierarchy emerges as a consequence of the nucleus or satellite of a relational schema being realised through spans rather than units. The hierarchy in rhetorical structure constitutes a "basic assumption underlying rhetorical structure analysis … that texts are not merely strings of clauses but are instead groups of hierarchically organized clauses which bear various informational and interactional relations to each other" (Fox 1987, p. 78). At the uppermost "macro level of organization" a single rhetorical relation governs the entire text (Stuart-Smith 2007, p. 42). For example, the text as a whole may constitute the answer to a problem posed in the title or narrate a story based on the title's theme. At the lowermost "local level of organization" one finds individual clause-to-clause relations, as illustrated in Figure 4.6 (Stuart-Smith 2007, p. 42). Since rhetorical structure analysis "describes how parts of a text combine through relations to make larger parts, which in turn combine to make up a whole text", one finds between the uppermost macro level of rhetorical governance and the lowermost local level of clause-to-clause relations "rhetorical 'chunking' of different text span sizes within a large text" (Stuart-Smith 2007, pp. 41–42). Each of these chunks (large spans) is governed by an overarching relation. Thus, as one progresses from the uppermost macro level of a text, down through the large spans comprising a text and ultimately down to the lowermost local level of clause-to-clause relations, a rhetorical hierarchy emerges.

In the sample texts' RST diagrams (Figure 4.7) this hierarchy of rhetorical governance is illustrated. The highest or 'primary' level of rhetorical governance of the text is signified by the overarching relation between the body of the text and the text title. Relations governing the largest spans (chunks) that make up the RST diagram of the body of a text constitute the 'secondary' level of rhetorical

(a) AUS Text 6:

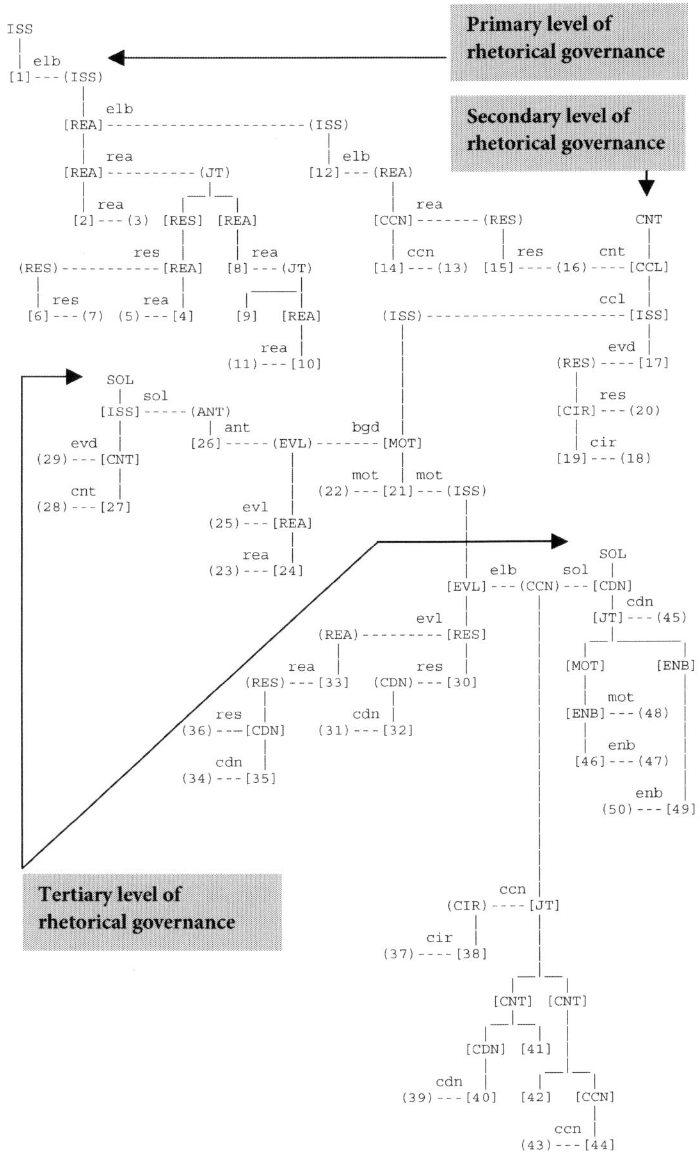

(b) PRC Text 3G:

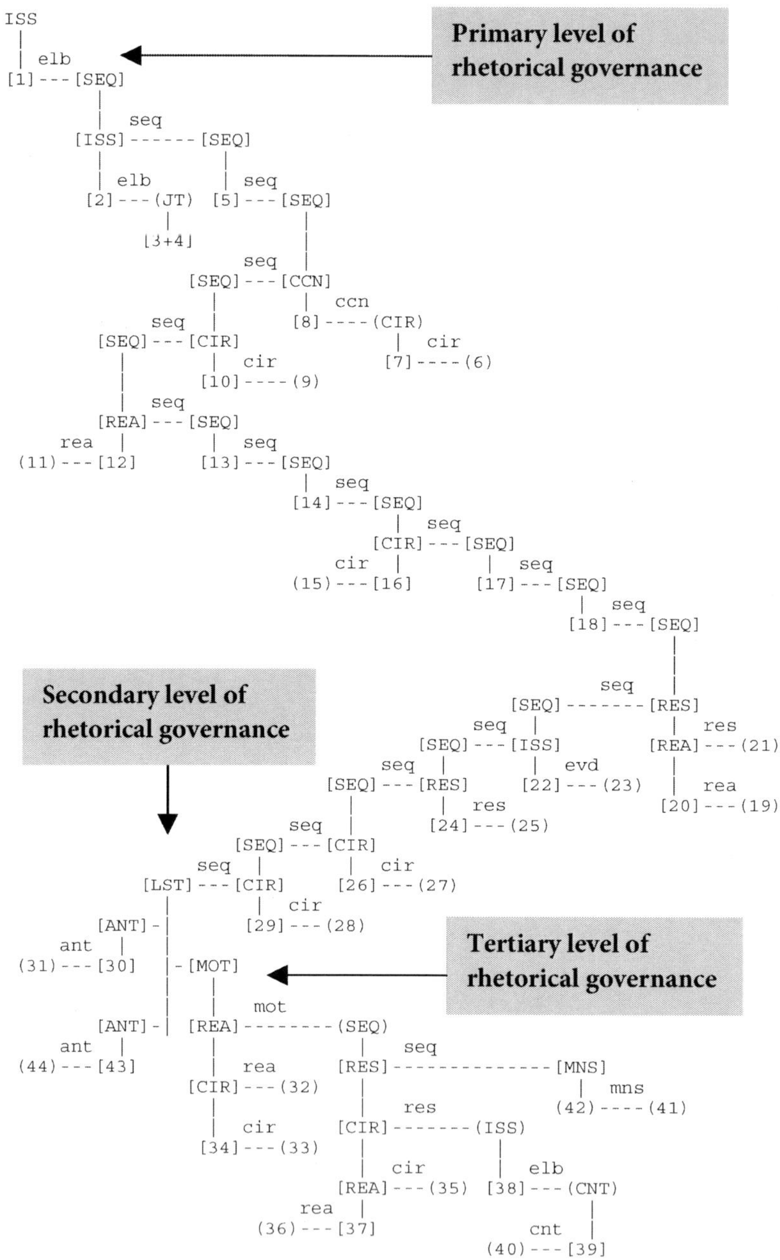
Primary level of rhetorical governance
Secondary level of rhetorical governance
Tertiary level of rhetorical governance

(c) TW Text 6 (extract)

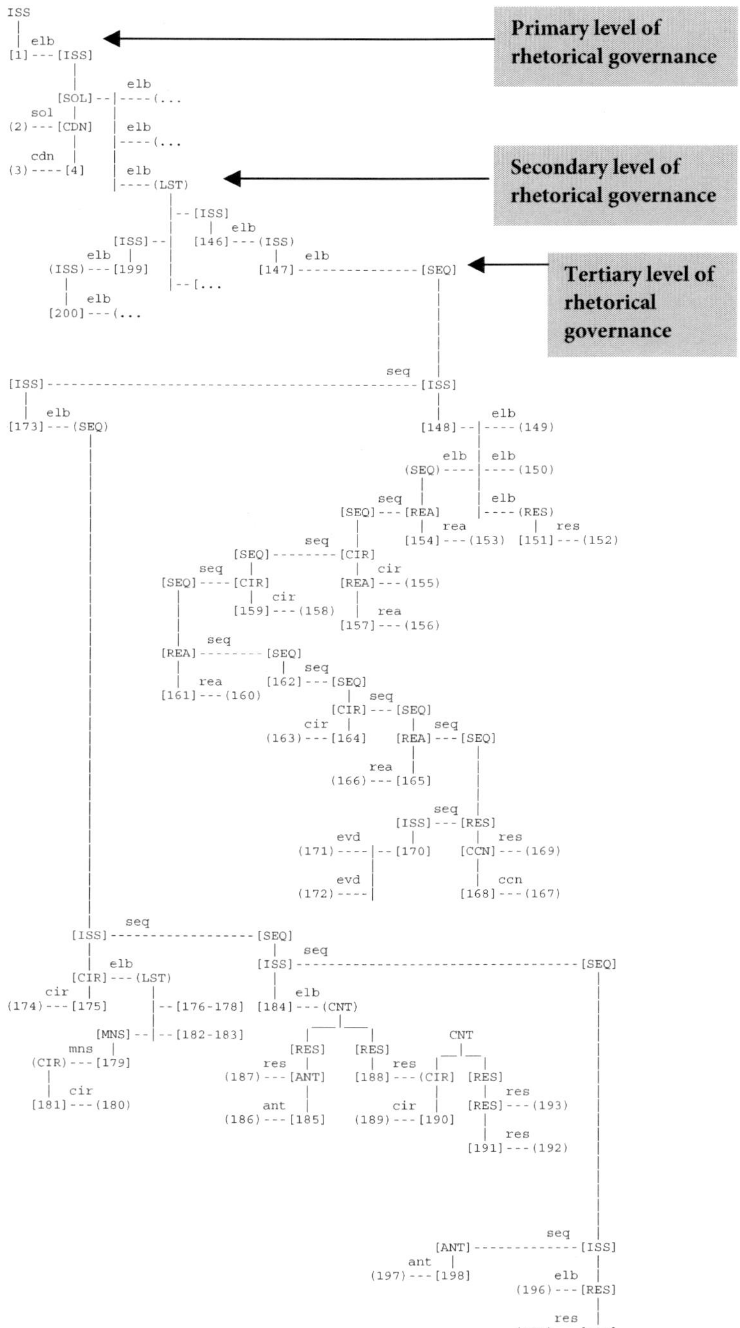

Figure 4.7. RST diagrams of sample texts

governance. These spans are comprised of a number of smaller spans, each governed by a relation ('tertiary' level of rhetorical governance). These higher levels of governance are of interest here, as they contribute to the dominant rhetorical form of a text, so levels of governance beyond the tertiary are not considered in this study.

Looking at the RST diagram for AUS Text 6 one finds at the primary level of rhetorical governance the elaboration relation (realised as an Issue schema). Thus, the body of the text (clause units 2–50) rhetorically constitutes an elaboration of the title, as opposed to, for example, the answer to a question posed in the title (Solution schema). At the secondary level of governance one finds a prominent Contrast schema governing two main spans covering clause units 2–16 and 17–50. Thus, within the main body of the text, the elicitation of comparison and difference can be considered as prominent in the rhetorical hierarchy. At the tertiary level of governance, that is, the smaller branching spans comprising the latter of the two main spans, Solution schema are most prominent. Thus, while solutions to problems feature rhetorically in AUS Text 6, they do so at a relatively lower level in the rhetorical hierarchy.

Looking at the RST diagram for PRC Text 3G one once again finds at the primary level of rhetorical governance the elaboration relation (realised as an Issue schema). Thus, the body of the text (clause units 2–44) rhetorically constitutes an elaboration of the title. Following a long sequential chain, at the secondary level of governance one finds a prominent List schema governing clause units 30–44. Most prominent in this list, at the tertiary level of governance, is a Motivation schema.

Looking at the RST diagram for TW Text 6 (extract) one again finds at the primary level of rhetorical governance the elaboration relation (realised as an Issue schema). Thus, the body of the text rhetorically constitutes an elaboration of the title. At the secondary level of governance one finds a prominent List schema governing an elaborative chain. Prominent in this chain, at the tertiary level of governance, is a Sequence schema.

The hierarchies of rhetorical governance of the three sample texts are illustrated in Figure 4.8.

Commenting on the hierarchy evident in RST diagrams, Abelen, Redeker and Thompson (1993, p. 339) state that "The highest levels of the rhetorical structure should most directly reflect the writer's overall purpose, while relations on lower levels can represent various subordinate goals". The upper levels of the hierarchy, therefore, embody the essential functions of a text, as presented to the reader. In AUS Text 6 this constitutes the provision of detail through a comparison of circumstances, culminating in the provision of solutions to deemed problems at

(a) AUS Text 6:

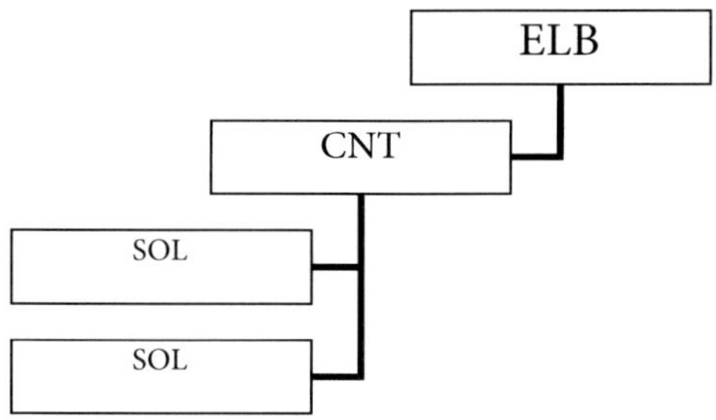

(b) PRC Text 3G:

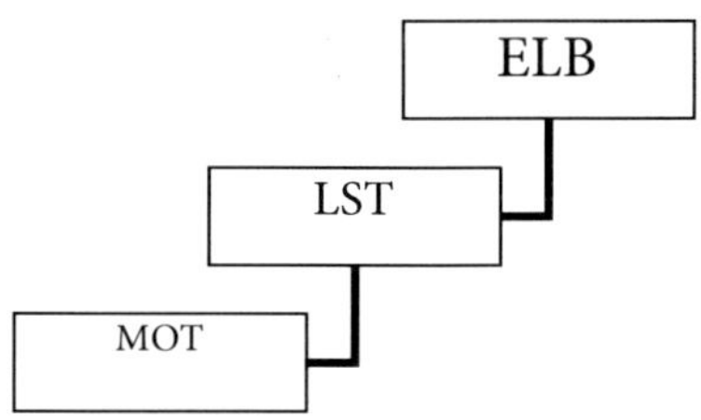

(c) TW Text 6 (extract):

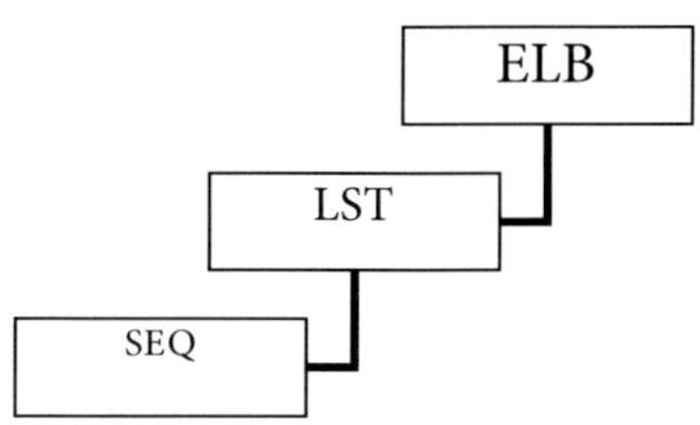

Figure 4.8 Hierarchy of rhetorical governance in sample texts

hand. In PRC Text 3G this constitutes the provision of detail, culminating in a list of recommendations with at least one playing a decidedly motivational role. In TW Text 6 (extract) this constitutes the provision of detail through the presentation of a series of narratives.

In addition to the representation of rhetorical hierarchy in a text, the RST diagram also allows quantification of the component rhetorical relations. The 'relative frequencies' of the relations comprising the three sample texts are presented in Figure 4.9.

(a) AUS Text 6:

Rhetorical relation	Number in RST diagram	Relative frequencies (rounded %)
ant	1	2
bgd	1	2
ccl	1	2
ccn	3	6.1
cdn	4	8.2
cir	2	4.1
cnt	4	8.2
elb	4	8.2
enb	2	4.1
evd	2	4.1
evl	2	4.1
jt	4	8.2
jus	0	0
lst	0	0
mns	0	0
mot	3	6.1
pur	0	0
rea	8	16.3
res	6	12.2
rtt	0	0
seq	0	0
sol	2	4.1
sum	0	0
TOTAL	49	100

(b) PRC Text 3G:

Rhetorical relation	Number in RST diagram	Relative frequencies (rounded %)
ant	2	4.8
bgd	0	0
ccl	0	0
ccn	1	2.4
cdn	0	0
cir	7	16.7
cnt	1	2.4
elb	3	7.1
enb	0	0
evd	1	2.4
evl	0	0

jt	1	2.4
jus	0	0
lst	1	2.4
mns	1	2.4
mot	1	2.4
pur	0	0
rea	4	9.5
res	3	7.1
rtt	0	0
seq	16	38.1
sol	0	0
sum	0	0
TOTAL	42	100

(c) TW Text 6 (extract):

Rhetorical relation	**Number in RST diagram**	**Relative frequencies (rounded %)**
ant	2	3.1
bgd	0	0
ccl	0	0
ccn	1	1.5
cdn	1	1.5
cir	6	9.2
cnt	2	3.1
elb	14	21.5
enb	0	0
evd	2	3.1
evl	0	0
jt	0	0
jus	0	0
lst	3	4.6
mns	1	1.5
mot	0	0
pur	0	0
rea	4	6.2
res	7	10.8
rtt	0	0
seq	21	32.3
sol	1	1.5
sum	0	0
TOTAL	65	100

Figure 4.9 Relative frequencies of sample texts' constituent rhetorical relations

Evaluation of text discursive form

Having a picture of a text's rhetorical makeup in terms of the relative frequencies of its functional relations and its hierarchy of rhetorical governance allows an analyst, in turn, to make determinations as to the discursive form of the text. This is because the rhetorical relations utilised in the RST framework suitably lend themselves to categorisations that reflect the discursive features of interest to a study. Such categorisations are purpose driven; there exists no exclusive taxonomy for the RST relations. Mann and Thompson, for example, have proposed a taxonomy distinguishing "subject matter" and "presentational" relations, whereby the former "serve mainly the purpose of information transfer" and the latter "aim at securing the reader's acceptance and collaboration" (Abelen, Redeker & Thompson 1993, p. 333). Abelen, Redeker and Thompson (1993, p. 323) subsequently drew on the classification of discourse functions proposed in systemic linguistics, broadening Mann and Thompson's taxonomy to incorporate "interpersonal, ideational, and textual" relations. Here, the ideational and textual "discourse relations" are seen to mediate "a greater concern with clarity" while the interpersonal mediate "open persuasion" (Abelen, Redeker & Thompson 1993, p. 323). Kong (1998) and Ramsay (2001b) provide other examples of RST relation taxonomies.

This study draws on the discursive 'voices' deemed salient to medical communication, as described in Chapter 3 of this volume, namely professional, institutional and client-centred, in order to categorise the rhetorical relations explicated in the psychoeducational texts. The resulting taxonomy is presented in Figure 4.10.

In this study, rhetorical relations signifying professional discourse encompass those mediating scientific expertise and specialised practice, in particular

Professional discourse	Institutional discourse	Client-centred discourse	Non-discourse-specific
conclusion	antithesis	background	joint
condition	concession	circumstance	
evidence	evaluation	contrast	
purpose	justification	elaboration	
reason	list	enablement	
result	motivation	means	
	restatement	sequence	
	solution		
	summary		

Figure 4.10 Taxonomy of rhetorical relations

the essential tenets of biomedicine (see Chapter 3, this volume). The emphasis here, therefore, is on the epistemological foundation to the practice of medicine, namely the science of biomedicine, its protocols and the world view it entails, as opposed to the utilitarian and pragmatic side to medical practice, such as maintaining authority and gaining patient compliance, which more reflect the institutional character of medical practice. Thus, in this study, rhetorical relations deemed to signify professional discourse (the professional voice of medicine) are as follows:

Reason, where cause is attributed; and result, as cause-and-effect or consequence (Noordman, Vonk & Simons 2000; Selander, et al. 1997).
由於這些藥物是不會令患者上癮的, 故此大部份精神分裂症患者都可以較全面再重投社會。 <Since these medications are not addictive, most people with schizophrenia can make a fairly complete return to society.> (AUS Text 4)
有時這些感受變得過強及持續很久， 以致人們很難處理或控制。 <Sometimes these feelings become overpowering and persist for a long time, such that people find it difficult to deal with or control.> (AUS Text 7)

Conclusion, where a position is logically deduced following a series of statements.
在澳洲, 社區服務可以給予你幫助。 你或需要金錢上的資助; 或需要短暫的休息, 使你有歇息的機會。 你不用單獨去處理全部的照顧。 <In Australia, community services can help you. You might need financial assistance or you might need temporary respite to give you the chance to take a rest. You do not need to deal with all the caregiving on your own.> (AUS Text 8)

Purpose, providing intention or rationale.
精神病患者在病情稳定后，需要重新学习生活、工作技能，以帮助他们更好地适应社会，增强自信心，回归社会生活。 <After their condition has stabilised, people with a mental illness need to re-learn life and work skills in order to help them better adapt to society, strengthen their self-confidence and return to life in society.> (PRC Text 1)

Condition, delimiting or qualifying through the unrealised or hypothetical.
如果及早察覺患上精神病, 就較易治療。 <If one is aware of mental illness early on then it is easier to treat.> (AUS Text 1)

Evidence, where a claim is substantiated.
精神病已不再是一种可怕及神秘的疾病，不少重性精神病患者都可透过服药、社区心理康复得到帮助，重投社会。 <Mental illness is no longer a frightening and mysterious disease. Many people with serious mental illness are able to return to society through taking medication and seeking psychological rehabilitation in the community.> (PRC Text 4)

Rhetorical relations signifying institutional discourse encompass those where authority is affirmed, those where consent is procured through coercive 'shouldness' and those that realise structural features characteristic of text produced by large organisations (see Chapter 3, this volume). The emphasis, therefore, is on those aspects of medical practice that reflect its authoritative basis, its wish to see professionally-determined outcomes achieved and the organisational requirement of structure, order and record-keeping. Thus, in this study, rhetorical relations deemed to signify institutional discourse (the institutional voice of medicine) are as follows:

Antithesis and Concession, where the correctness of a preferred viewpoint is affirmed to the exclusion or subordination of an alternative. With Antithesis, an alternative perspective or compromise is refuted or denied.
这时,切不可简单粗暴地批评、指责病人,而应以宽容的态度善待他们。 <At these times, you simply cannot gruffly criticise and find fault with the ill person, but should treat them kindly in a tolerant way.> (PRC Text 2)

With Concession, while an alternative perspective may be proffered, giving the appearance of conciliation or compromise, this alternative in the end is subordinated to a preferred position. As such, Azar (1999, p. 106) states, "presentation of a counter-argument" in a concession relation is "psychologically manipulative" in that "such a maneuver … eliminates a possible unfavorable intervention and also reinforces the credibility of the [preferred position], because the readers are led to understand that the writer has already considered [alternative perspectives] … and rejected them." Thus, the pre-eminence of the authoritative position is maintained.
这些药物亦可能引致一些令人不适的副作用，但这些副作用是有办法减少的。 <These medications might also lead to some unpleasant side effects, but there are ways to reduce these side effects.> (PRC Text 4)

Justification, where an unqualified right to advance a position is asserted, usually relating to an authoritative position or professional experience.
那种认为结婚可为病人"冲喜"，使疾病好转的说法是极端错误的，没有科学根据。
<That kind of way of thinking that says marriage can bring happiness to the ill person and cause the disease to change for the better is extremely mistaken. It has no scientific basis.> (PRC Text 2)

Evaluation, where authority is presumed to proffer positive or negative commentary that tends to advance a preferred viewpoint. While Evaluation may be integral to the protocol of any professional intercession or assessment, or may give the appearance of consumer engagement or input, at the core of the evaluation relation is a presumed entitlement or privilege to make an assessment. This presumption both stems from and maintains the authoritative position.
康复者需要家庭温暖，家人的亲情和关爱至为重要。 <The person in recovery needs a warm family environment. A family's love and care are very important.> (PRC Text 5)

Motivation and Solution, where consent is procured through grades of coercion ('shouldness'), ranging from the covert to the overt. Motivation utilises incentive to draw one toward a preferred position or practice ('you should do this as you will get this reward'), while Solution uncompromisingly provides *the* answer to a problem or question ('this is what you should do').
患有這些症狀的人應尋求醫務人員的幫助。。。患者在剛生病時或病情加劇前接受治療，就有可能較快地康復。 <People with these symptoms should seek help from medical personnel … If sufferers receive treatment when they have just fallen ill or before their condition intensifies then a more speedy recovery is possible.> (AUS Text 2)

腦部的化學不平衡可以引致憂鬱症，這個問題或可以抗憂鬱藥物來治理。 <Imbalance of chemicals in the brain can lead to depression. This problem may be controlled by anti-depressive medication.> (AUS Text 5)

Restatement, frequently used as a persuasive strategy or to call attention to an issue, particularly in political and marketing discourse.
憂鬱是什麼？ 憂鬱是什麼？ 須先認識「憂鬱情緒」與「憂鬱症」的差別。 <**What is depression?** What is depression? One first needs to know the difference between "depressed mood" and "clinical depression".> (TW Text 5)

List and Summary, which tend to feature structurally in texts produced by large organisations.
以下任何症狀都可能與抑鬱症相關：
- 感到憂鬱, 易哭
- 睡眠不安
- 食慾與體重變化
- 失去興趣與動力

<Any of the following symptoms could be related to depression:
- feeling depressed and crying easily
- restless sleep
- change in appetite and body weight
- loss of interest in things and motivation> (AUS Text 3)

… 總之, 精神病人慢性化的過程中, 一方面需要家人付出更多的關心、耐心、了解和幫忙, 另一方面要和醫療機構配合, 定期門診治療及參加復健。 <… In short, the chronic course of disease for the person with a mental illness requires, on the one hand, greater care, patience, understanding and help from the family and, on the other hand, cooperation with health agencies, regular outpatient treatment and participating in rehabilitation.> (TW Text 7)

Rhetorical relations signifying client-centredness encompass those mediating consumer empowerment, active choice and the recounting of life experience (see Chapter 3, this volume). In this study, rhetorical relations deemed to signify client-centred discourse (the client-centred voice) are as follows:

Background, circumstance, elaboration and means, where context and detail are proffered.
我于1982年不幸患精神分裂症，带病考上并读完大学，至今一直服维持量 。。。
我生活在一个橱子里，它不像一般的橱子，无人能看见它、摸到它，或到里面来陪伴我。
<In 1982 I had the misfortune to develop schizophrenia. In spite of the illness I passed the university entrance exam and completed my university studies. To date I have remained on a maintenance dose of medication …
I live in a closet. It is not like a regular closet: nobody can see it, touch it or accompany me inside it.> (PRC Text 3)
在數次的就醫過程中，不論花費多昂貴、需要多少的時間做治療，阿公都不放棄任何能讓阿嬤病情好起來的方法。 <In the process of seeing the doctor many times, no matter how expensive the cost or how much time was required for treatment, Grandad never gave up on any means for making Grandma's condition better.> (TW Text 6)
我是1991年10月成为一名精神病患者的，那时我刚刚大学毕业，踏上工作岗位仅仅一个星期。 <I developed a mental illness in October 1991. At the time, I had only just graduated from university and had set foot in my workplace for barely a week.> (PRC Text 3)

母亲经过自我反省和多方的辅导后，明白到自己纵有不足之处，但仍是一位称职的母亲。 <Through soul-searching and many forms of counselling Mother came to understand that even if there were some shortcomings she remained a capable mother.> (PRC Text 5)

Contrast, where choice, options and comparisons are volunteered.
不但原来的症状没去掉，反而添了其他症状。 <Not only did the original symptoms not abate, but on the contrary other symptoms emerged.> (PRC Text 3)

Enablement, where the realisation of an action is made possible.
照護員協會可替你聯絡當地的華籍社區工作員、照護員支持小組、專業人士及義工服務。你可以隨時致電給他們 。。。 照護員協會電話列於第三頁。 <The carers' association can get in touch with the local Chinese community workers, carers' support group and specialist and volunteer services on your behalf. You can phone them at any time … The carers' association's telephone number is listed on page three.> (AUS Text 8)

Sequence (narrative), where events are recounted in a temporally coherent sequence (story) (He 1998). Gwyn (2002, p. 140) notes that "it is … sequentiality which differentiates narrative from other forms of conveying and apprehending information."
当时我感到莫名其妙, 忍不住失声痛哭。 妈妈也只是给我做了非常简单的解释：“爸爸不能看电视。” 我的心里非常难过。 <At the time I felt bewildered and could not help but weep involuntarily. Mummy only gave me a very simple explanation: "Daddy is not up to watching television." In my heart I was extremely upset.> (PRC Text 3)

The joint relation, equating to a rhetorical conjunction, is classified as non-discourse-specific in that it is not distinctive of any of the salient discourses in question.

Applying Figure 4.10's categorisations to the three sample texts, the texts' relative discursive compositions, as calculated from the relative frequencies in Figure 4.9, are illustrated below (Figure 4.11).

In Figure 4.12, percentages adjusted for the discursive non-specificity of the joint relation provide a measure of the 'discursive content' of the text (see Chapter 3, this volume).

Thus, proportionally, the professional voice of medicine dominates the AUS sample text and the client-centred voice dominates the PRC and TW sample texts in virtually equal manner.

Figure 4.13 illustrates the discursive hierarchies of the three sample texts, based on the hierarchy of rhetorical governance presented in Figure 4.8.

Combining the findings of Figures 4.12 and 4.13, AUS Text 6 presents as client-centred in discursive form, yet a greater proportion of the text resonates the professional voice of medicine. On the other hand, a greater proportion of PRC Text 3G and the extract of TW Text 6 resonates the client-centred voice (specifically the 'lifeworld voice' of narrative), despite the prominence of institutional features in their upper-level discursive hierarchies. The Australian sample text,

(a) AUS Text 6:

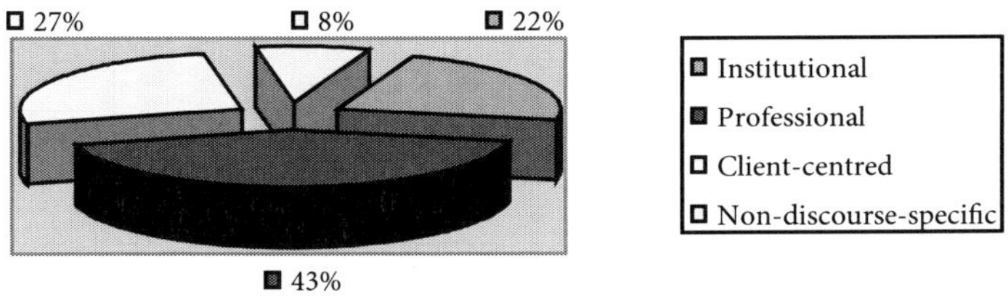

(b) PRC Text 3G:

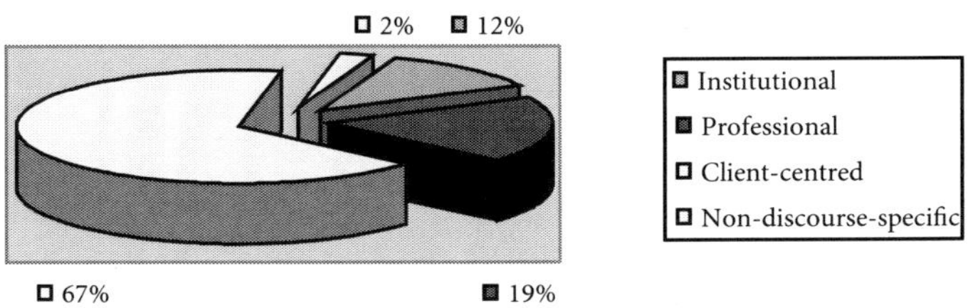

(c) TW Text 6 (extract):

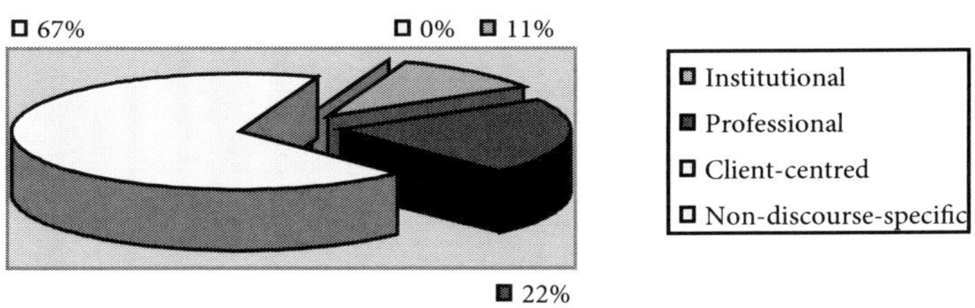

Figure 4.11 Relative discursive composition of sample texts

therefore, appears to discursively present to its reader as engaging and empowering (client-centred) while its discursive core remains characteristically biomedical in form (cf. the outward 'conversationalisation' of institutional communication in the West, noted in Chapter 3 of this volume). The PRC and Taiwanese sample texts, on the other hand, are seemingly more visibly marked as institutional in form yet their discursive cores draw heavily on the lifeworld.

In subsequent sections, the analytic findings for the three corpora of psycho-educational texts under study (PRC, Taiwanese and Australian) are presented in like manner.

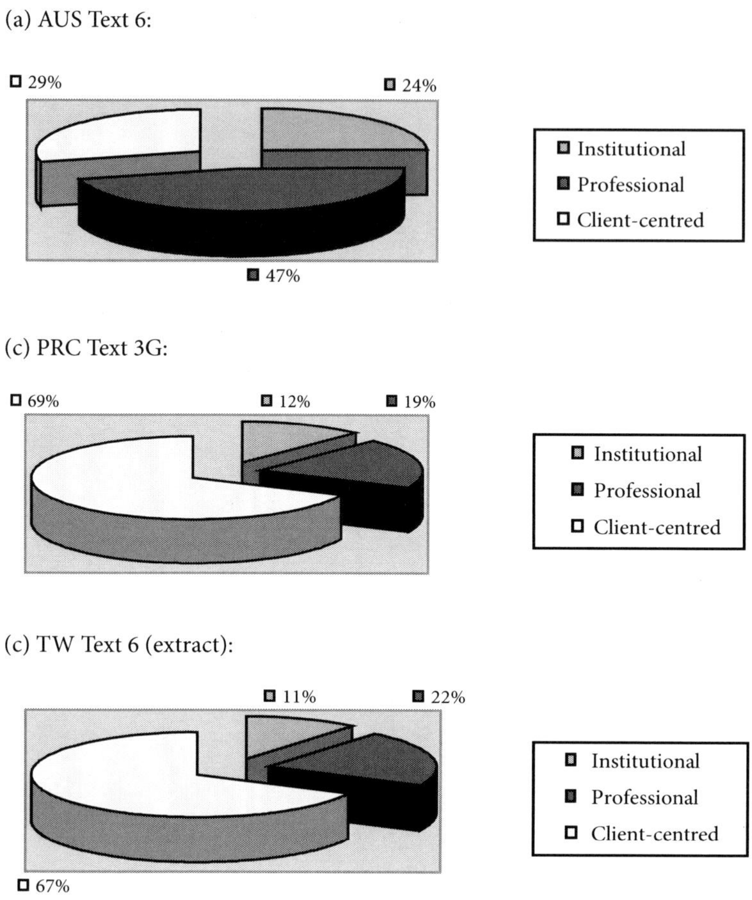

Figure 4.12 Discursive content of sample texts (adjusted for joint relation)

Analytic findings for mainland Chinese psychoeducational literature

The corpus of mainland Chinese (PRC) psychoeducational texts analysed in this study is drawn from a body of literature collected during a field trip to mainland China during the months of December and January of 2002–2003. It was obtained from hospitals and non-government mental health bodies in Beijing (northern China) and Guangzhou (southern China). Literature was collected from both regions in light of the geographical vastness of mainland China and the potential differences that could emerge as a consequence of southern China's

(a) AUS Text 6:

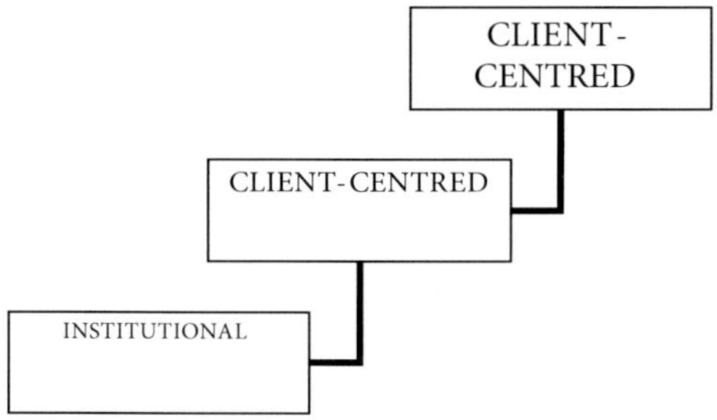

(b) PRC Text 3G:

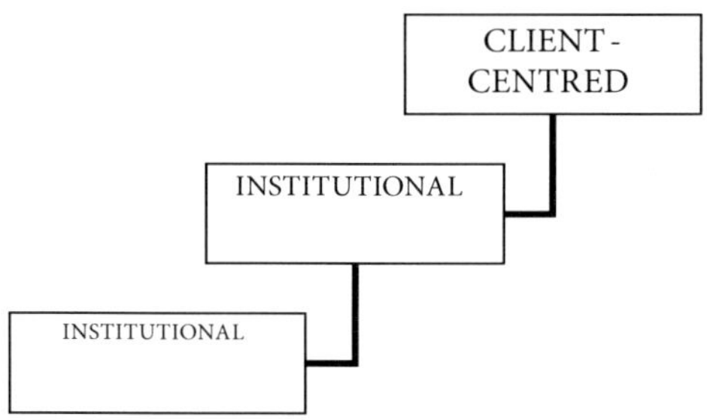

(c) TW Text 6 (extract):

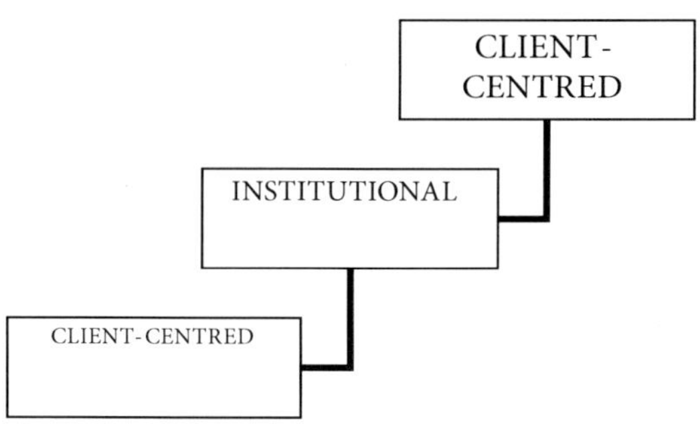

Figure 4.13 Discursive hierarchies of sample texts

distance from the seat of central government in Beijing and its proximity to the former British colony of Hong Kong. Indeed, the southern literature was produced by the Likang Family Resource Centre in Guangzhou, a joint project of the Richmond Fellowship of Hong Kong and the Guangzhou Federation for the Disabled, which provides services to people with a mental illness and their carers in the Guangzhou district. Authorship of the PRC literature was limited, with just three sources dominating: the China Disabled Persons' Federation, the Likang Family Resource Centre and the Mental Health Research Institute of Beijing University (Yao Guizhong).

The PRC psychoeducational texts were lengthy, limiting the number of texts comprising the PRC corpus to five. The five texts were chosen on the following bases:

1. Topic. By and large the PRC texts deal with mental illness generically, with only one sourced text focusing on specific illness. Accordingly, four texts selected for analysis deal with mental illness generically, with one text (Text 1) dealing specifically with psychotic mental illness.
2. Form of publication. The PRC texts came in the form of tri-fold pamphlet, booklet, newsletter and edited monograph. Each form was represented amongst the five texts selected. In the case of the psychoeducational newsletter and edited monograph (itself a compilation of newsletter texts), due to excessive length, representative texts comprising these publications (mostly personal and carer narratives about mental illness) were drawn and analysed individually. The results of the analysis of the individual texts drawn from each publication are combined as PRC Text(s) 3 and PRC Text(s) 5.
3. Place of publication. Reflecting the relative numbers of sourced texts, the corpus contains three texts of northern origin (Beijing) and two of southern origin (Guangzhou).

Details of the texts selected for study are listed in Figure 4.14.

The relative frequencies of rhetorical relations for each of these texts and the average for all PRC texts analysed are presented in Figure 4.15. On average, elaboration (16.7%) followed by sequence (9.6%) relations constitute the larger proportions of the analysed PRC psychoeducational literature. Individually, however, sequence relations dominate only Text(s) 3 (31.3%) and Text(s) 5 (14.7%), where narrative is extensively utilised. Sequence relations do not feature strongly in the other PRC texts. Text 1, dealing with psychotic mental illness, has well above average levels of antithesis relations (12.1%). Restatement, summary, justification and enablement relations are minimal both on average and within individual texts.

Figure 4.16 illustrates the proportional discursive content of each text as well as the average for all PRC texts analysed. Client-centred discourse features substantially in all the PRC psychoeducational texts, as the proportionally largest or essentially equal largest discursive presence. Taken as an average, client-centred discourse eclipses the professional and the institutional; nevertheless, it does not constitute a majority (> 50%). It is interesting to note that despite their

	TEXT 1	TEXT 2	TEXT(S) 3	TEXT 4	TEXT(S) 5
Title	消除偏见勇于关爱 (Do away with discrimination and have the courage to care)	你知道吗？ (Did you know?)	精神疾病康复文集 (Selected readings on recovery from mental illness)	认识精神病小册子 (Getting to know mental illness)	利康通讯 (Likang newsletter)
Author / publisher	中国残疾人联合会 (China Disabled Persons' Federation)	中国残疾人联合会 (China Disabled Persons' Federation)	姚贵忠主编 / 中国科学技术出版社 (Yao Guizhong Chief Editor /China Science & Technology Press)	利康家属资源中心 (Likang Family Resource Centre)	利康家属资源中心 (Likang Family Resource Centre)
Year of publication	c2002	c2002	2000	2000	2002
Place of publication	Beijing, PRC	Beijing, PRC	Beijing, PRC	Guangzhou, PRC	Guangzhou, PRC
Description	Glossy tri-fold pamphlet	8 page glossy booklet	451 page edited monograph	23 page plain paper booklet	Edited newsletter (2 issues – one 8 page, one 10 page)
Topic	Mental illness – psychosis	Mental Illness – general	Mental illness – general	Mental illness – general	Mental illness – general

Figure 4.14 Identification details of PRC psychoeducational texts

Relations	TEXT 1		TEXT 2		TEXT(S) 3		TEXT 4		TEXT(S) 5		PRC text average
	nos	%(rnd)	nos	%(rnd)	nos	%(rnd)	nos	%(rnd)	nos	%(rnd)	%(rnd)
ant	8	12.1	2	1	7	1.5	8	1.8	5	3.7	4
bgd	4	6.1	3	1.5	9	1.9	15	3.4	1	0.7	2.7
ccl	1	1.5	2	1	6	1.3	6	1.4	3	2.2	1.5
ccn	4	6.1	5	2.5	34	7.3	25	5.7	8	5.9	5.5
cdn	5	7.6	13	6.4	15	3.2	17	3.9	3	2.2	4.7
cir	7	10.6	19	9.4	32	6.9	22	5	8	5.9	7.6
cnt	3	4.5	9	4.5	22	4.7	9	2.1	2	1.5	3.5
elb	6	9.1	47	23.3	49	10.5	140	32	12	8.8	16.7
enb	1	1.5	3	1.5	0	0	1	0.2	0	0	0.6
evd	8	12.1	6	3	34	7.3	14	3.2	19	14	7.9
evl	1	1.5	3	1.5	20	4.3	4	0.9	11	8.1	3.3
jt	1	1.5	7	3.5	10	2.1	23	5.3	5	3.7	3.2
jus	0	0	1	0.5	0	0	0	0	0	0	0.1
lst	1	1.5	17	8.4	2	0.4	21	4.8	2	1.5	3.3
mns	3	4.5	11	5.4	2	0.4	4	0.9	3	2.2	2.7
mot	1	1.5	11	5.4	6	1.3	26	5.9	9	6.6	4.1
pur	1	1.5	4	2	9	1.9	11	2.5	7	5.1	2.6
rea	1	1.5	8	4	26	5.6	11	2.5	5	3.7	3.5
res	9	13.6	16	7.9	27	5.8	28	6.4	9	6.6	8.1
rtt	0	0	0	0	0	0	0	0	0	0	0
seq	0	0	1	0.5	146	31.3	6	1.4	20	14.7	9.6
sol	1	1.5	14	6.9	11	2.4	47	10.7	4	2.9	4.9
sum	0	0	0	0	0	0	0	0	0	0	0
TOTAL	66	100	202	100	467	100	438	100	136	100	100

Figure 4.15 Relative frequencies in PRC psychoeducational texts

high proportion of sequence (narrative) relations, PRC Texts 3 and 5 in the end are not set apart from their counterparts discursively; in fact they represent the polar extremes of client-centredness (56% & 35%, respectively). This is because the narrative presence in Text 5 is offset by a substantial presence of professional discourse (mediated in particular by the evidence relation), thus diminishing the degree of client-centredness. Text 1 that addresses psychotic mental illness most strongly resonates the professional voice of medicine (38%). These issues will be taken up in Chapter 5.

Figure 4.17 compares the discursive composition of psychoeducational texts sourced from northern and southern regions of the PRC. This comparison is undertaken due to Guangzhou's close proximity to Hong Kong, which remained

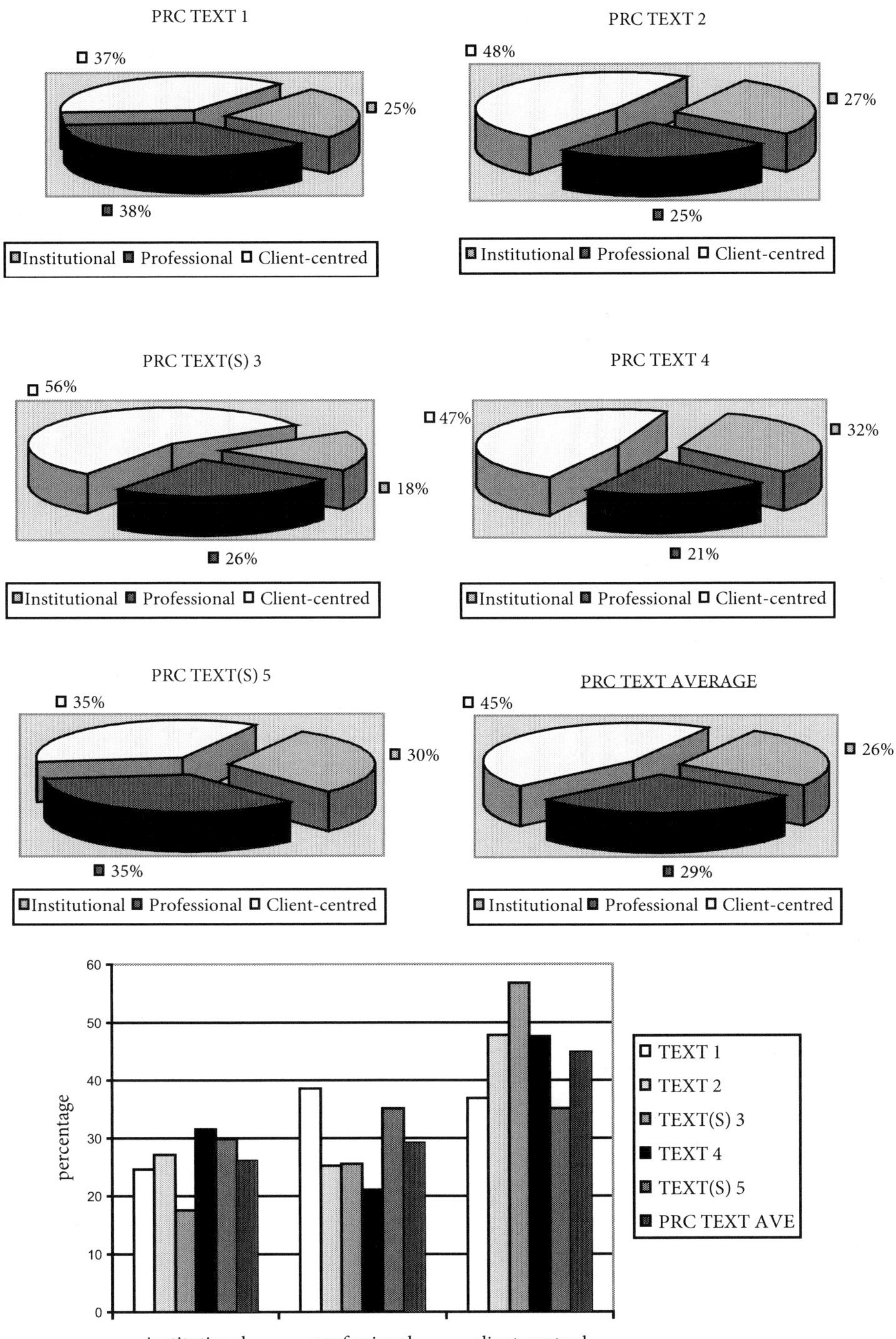

Figure 4.16 Discursive content of PRC psychoeducational texts

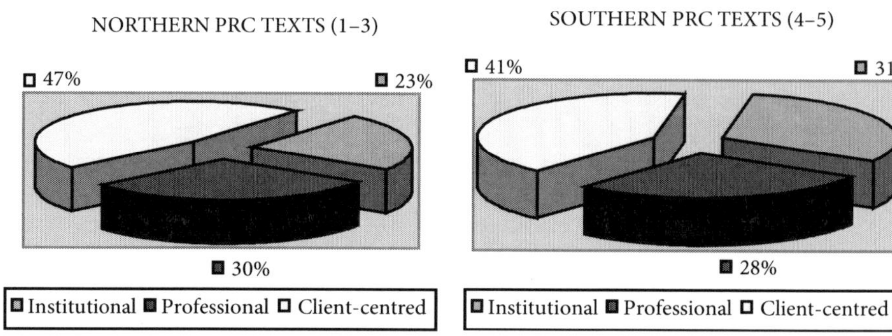

Figure 4.17 Discursive content of PRC psychoeducational texts by region

under British colonial rule from the 1840s until its return to China in 1997. As a consequence of the longstanding British presence, Western attitudes could possibly have gained a foothold in Hong Kong mental health circles. Given that the Guangzhou psychoeducational texts under study are produced by a joint Hong Kong and Guangzhou undertaking, the Likang Family Resource Centre, there is a need to determine if any Western-derived Hong Kong influences distinguish the southern PRC literature from its northern counterparts.

While texts from the two regions are equally professional in discursive content, the northern PRC psychoeducational texts are more client-centred and less institutional than the southern texts. In order to further explore this regional difference, comparisons need to be made with findings obtained from the Taiwanese and Australian corpora (see Chapter 5, this volume).

Figure 4.18 illustrates the discursive hierarchies of the PRC psychoeducational texts and the PRC text average. Typically, client-centredness is found at the highest level of the discursive hierarchy, with institutional forms dominating the penultimate levels. The PRC texts with a high narrative element (Texts 3 & 5), however, are not dominated by institutional forms at any level, with client-centredness dominating the primary level and a scattering of discursive forms evident in secondary and tertiary levels. Regionally, while client-centredness dominates the highest level of the southern texts' hierarchies, in the northern texts client-centred *and* institutional forms equally dominate. The potential significance of these differences will be further discussed in Chapter 5.

In sum, analysis of the PRC psychoeducational texts has revealed a literature that is appreciably client-centred. When regional differences are taken into account, a picture emerges whereby southern texts present as client-centred with institutional features at penultimate levels of governance. They display proportionally more institutional content than northern texts. The latter, in contrast,

(a) Discursive hierarchies of PRC psychoeducational texts

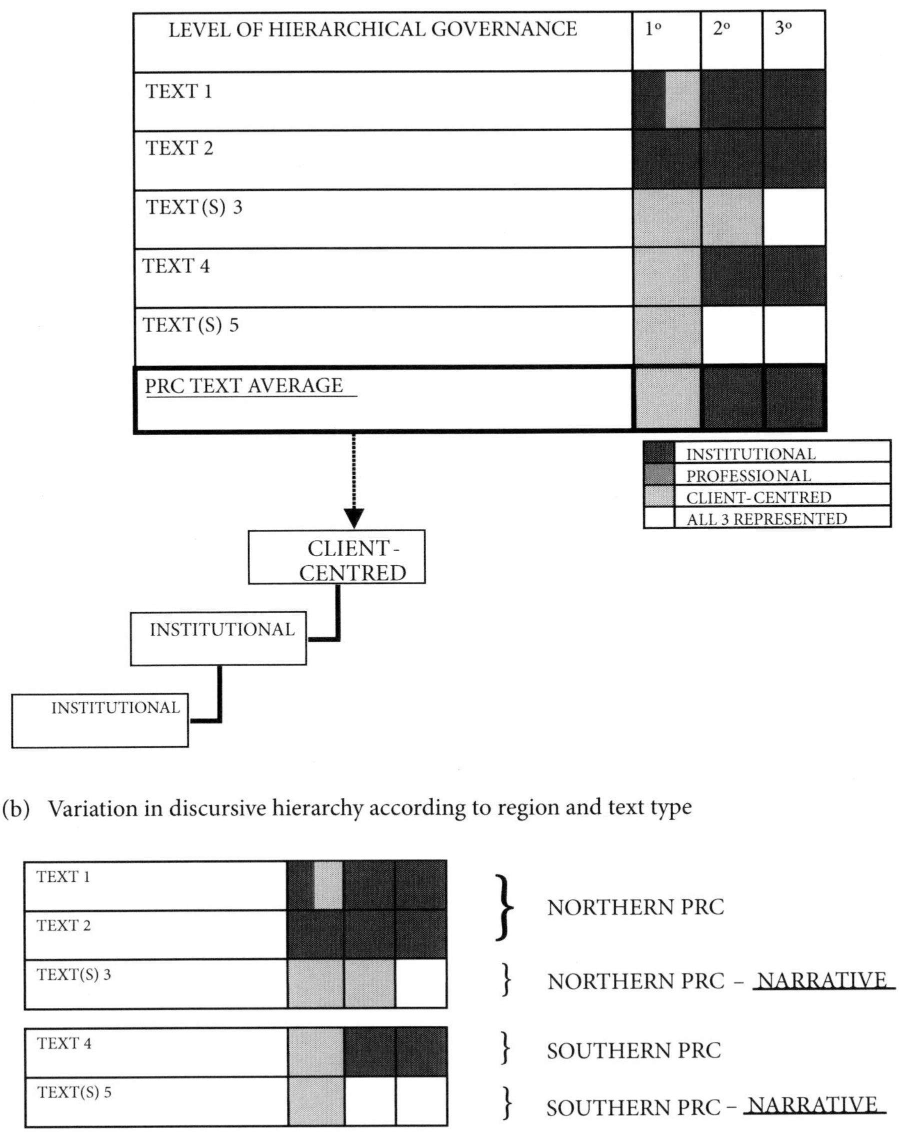

Figure 4.18

generally are more institutional in presentation but proportionally more client-centred in discursive content.

Analytic findings for the Taiwanese psychoeducational literature

The corpus of Taiwanese (TW) psychoeducational literature analysed in this study is drawn from a body of literature collected during a field trip to Taiwan during March 2005. Like the PRC corpus, the literature was obtained from hospitals and non-government mental health bodies, in this case, located in the Taipei district. As a small island, regional differences were not considered of concern here. Authorship of the TW literature was once again limited, with three sources dominating: the Taipei City Psychiatric Center, the John Tung Foundation and the Department of Health of the Executive Yuan of the Republic of China (Taiwan).

The TW psychoeducational texts were not as lengthy as their PRC counterparts, allowing slightly more individual texts (seven) to be analysed. The seven texts were chosen on the following bases:

1. Topic. While once again focussing on mental illness generically, in the sourced TW literature there were more publications dealing with specific illness (depression more so than schizophrenia), as compared to the PRC literature. There were also more publications examining caregiving and pharmacotherapy in mental illness. Accordingly, texts were chosen for analysis to reflect this spread of topics.
2. Form of publication. The TW texts came in the form of tri-fold pamphlet, brochure and monograph. Each form was represented amongst the five texts selected. In the case of the psychoeducational monograph, due to its length, only the chapter dealing with schizophrenia was analysed. Schizophrenia was preferentially chosen due to the lack of attention to the illness in any other publication form.

Details of the texts selected for study are listed in Figure 4.19.

The relative frequencies of rhetorical relations for each of these texts and the average for all TW texts analysed are presented in Figure 4.20. On average, elaboration (26.6%) comprises the larger proportion of the analysed TW psychoeducational literature. While sequence relations are less evident compared to the PRC result, TW Text 5 (9.9%) and Text 6 (18.8%) individually attain the PRC average. Like their PRC counterparts, both feature narrative and, interestingly, both deal solely with the issue of clinical depression. Text 1, dealing with treatment options, has a well above average level of purpose relations (11.0%) and Text 3, dealing

	TEXT 1	TEXT 2	TEXT 3	TEXT 4
Title	精神疾病的治療模式 (Modes of treatment for mental illness)	認識精神病 (Getting to know mental illness)	慢性精神病患的生活適應與照顧 (Lifestyle adjustments and care for people with chronic mental illness)	家人罹患心理疾病 (Family members suffering from mental illness)
Author / publisher	台北市立療養院 (Taipei City Psychiatric Center)	台北市立療養院 (Taipei City Psychiatric Center)	台北市立療養院 (Taipei City Psychiatric Center)	Channing Bete Co., South Deerfield, MA., U.S.A. Translated by 台北市立療養院 (Taipei City Psychiatric Center)
Year of publication	2001	c2000	1990	1986
Place of publication	Taipei, RoC (TW)	Taipei, RoC	Taipei, RoC	Taipei, RoC
Description	Glossy tri-fold pamphlet	Glossy tri-fold pamphlet	Glossy tri-fold pamphlet	12 page plain paper brochure
Topic	Mental illness – therapy	Mental Illness – general	Mental Illness – caregiving	Mental illness – general

	TEXT 5	TEXT 6	TEXT 7
Title	憂鬱，不只是想太多 (Depression is not just about thinking too much)	走出憂鬱迎向藍天 (Walk out of depression and into clear skies)	如何幫助精神病人: 認識精神病 (How to help people with a mental illness: getting to know mental illness)
Author / publisher	財團法人董氏基金會 (John Tung Foundation)	財團法人董氏基金會 (John Tung Foundation)	行政院衛生署 (Department of Health, Executive Yuan, RoC)
Year of publication	2001	c2000	c2000
Place of publication	Taipei, RoC	Taipei, RoC	Taipei, RoC
Description	20 page colour brochure	17 page colour brochure	50 page monograph
Topic	Depression	Depression	Mental illness – general & schizophrenia

Figure 4.19 Identification details of TW psychoeducational texts

with caring for people with a mental illness, has a well above average level of enablement relations (5.6%). As with the PRC texts, restatement, summary and justification relations are minimal both on average and within individual texts. With the exception of Text 3 mentioned above, levels of enablement relations in the TW texts are low.

Relations	TEXT 1		TEXT 2		TEXT 3		TEXT 4		TEXT 5	
	nos	%(rnd)	nos	%(rnd)	nos	%(rnd)	nos	%(rnd)	nos	%(rnd)
ant	1	1.2	4	7.5	3	4.2	13	7.6	9	4.2
bgd	1	1.2	0	0	1	1.4	1	1	6	2.8
ccl	0	0	1	1.9	0	0	0	0	3	1.4
ccn	0	0	2	3.8	0	0	5	3	9	4.2
cdn	0	0	0	0	4	5.6	9	5	12	5.6
cir	8	9.8	2	3.8	7	9.7	8	5	18	8.5
cnt	0	0	0	0	2	2.8	0	0	12	5.6
elb	32	39	17	32.1	14	19.4	45	26	49	23
enb	0	0	0	0	4	5.6	6	3	1	0.5
evd	3	3.7	10	18.9	4	5.6	9	5	2	0.9
evl	1	1.2	1	1.9	0	0	4	2	2	0.9
jt	3	3.7	0	0	1	1.4	4	2	10	4.7
jus	0	0	0	0	0	0	0	0	0	0
lst	10	12.2	4	7.5	6	8.3	18	10	8	3.8
mns	1	1.2	1	1.9	1	1.4	4	2	1	0.5
mot	1	1.2	4	7.5	3	4.2	8	5	5	2.3
pur	9	11	1	1.9	2	2.8	10	6	4	1.9
rea	2	2.4	1	1.9	3	4.2	6	3	9	4.2
res	4	4.9	3	5.7	8	11.1	8	5	12	5.6
rtt	0	0	0	0	0	0	0	0	1	0.5
seq	1	1.2	0	0	4	5.6	0	0	21	9.9
sol	5	6.1	2	3.8	5	6.9	14	8	19	8.9
sum	0	0	0	0	0	0	0	0	0	0
TOTAL	82	100	53	100	72	100	172	100	213	100

Relations	TEXT 6		TEXT 7		TW text average
	nos	%(rnd)	nos	%(rnd)	%(rnd)
ant	9	3.4	8	3.1	4.5
bgd	1	0.4	6	2.3	1.3
ccl	5	1.9	1	0.4	0.8
ccn	15	5.7	12	4.7	3.1
cdn	13	5	23	8.9	4.3
cir	23	8.8	13	5.1	7.2

cnt	8	3.1	10	3.9	2.2
elb	57	21.8	64	24.9	26.6
enb	5	1.9	1	0.4	1.6
evd	8	3.1	9	3.5	5.8
evl	2	0.8	3	1.2	1.1
jt	5	1.9	4	1.6	2.2
jus	0	0	0	0	0
lst	7	2.7	5	1.9	6.6
mns	3	1.1	3	1.2	1.3
mot	2	0.8	6	2.3	3.3
pur	4	1.5	13	5.1	4.3
rea	18	6.9	17	6.6	4.2
res	14	5.4	31	12.1	7.1
rtt	0	0	0	0	0.1
seq	49	18.8	9	3.5	5.6
sol	17	6.5	18	7	6.7
sum	0	0	1	0.4	0.1
TOTAL	265	100	257	100	100

Figure 4.20 Relative frequencies in TW psychoeducational texts

Figure 4.21 illustrates the proportional discursive content of each text as well as the average for all TW texts analysed. As with the PRC literature, client-centred discourse features substantially in all the TW psychoeducational texts, as the proportionally largest discursive presence. Taken as an average, client-centred discourse again eclipses the professional and the institutional, yet does not constitute a majority (> 50%). Of particular interest here are the disease-specific texts: Texts 5 and 6 dealing with clinical depression, which both display a very high degree of client-centredness (53% & 56%, respectively); in contrast to Text 7 which addresses schizophrenia, where the professional voice of medicine resonates at a level well above that found in any other text (37%).

Most of the TW psychoeducational texts are analogous to their northern PRC counterparts in that they are decidedly client-centred and less institutional in composition. However, two texts (Texts 2 & 4) stand out, possessing notably higher institutional values (32% & 37%, respectively), reminiscent of the southern PRC texts. Interestingly, Text 4 originates from the United States. This issue will be further explored in the Chapter 5.

Figure 4.22 illustrates the discursive hierarchies of the TW psychoeducational texts and the TW text average. Like the PRC literature, typically, client-centredness is found at the highest level of the discursive hierarchy, with the institutional voice governing penultimate levels. A minority of texts have institutional forms

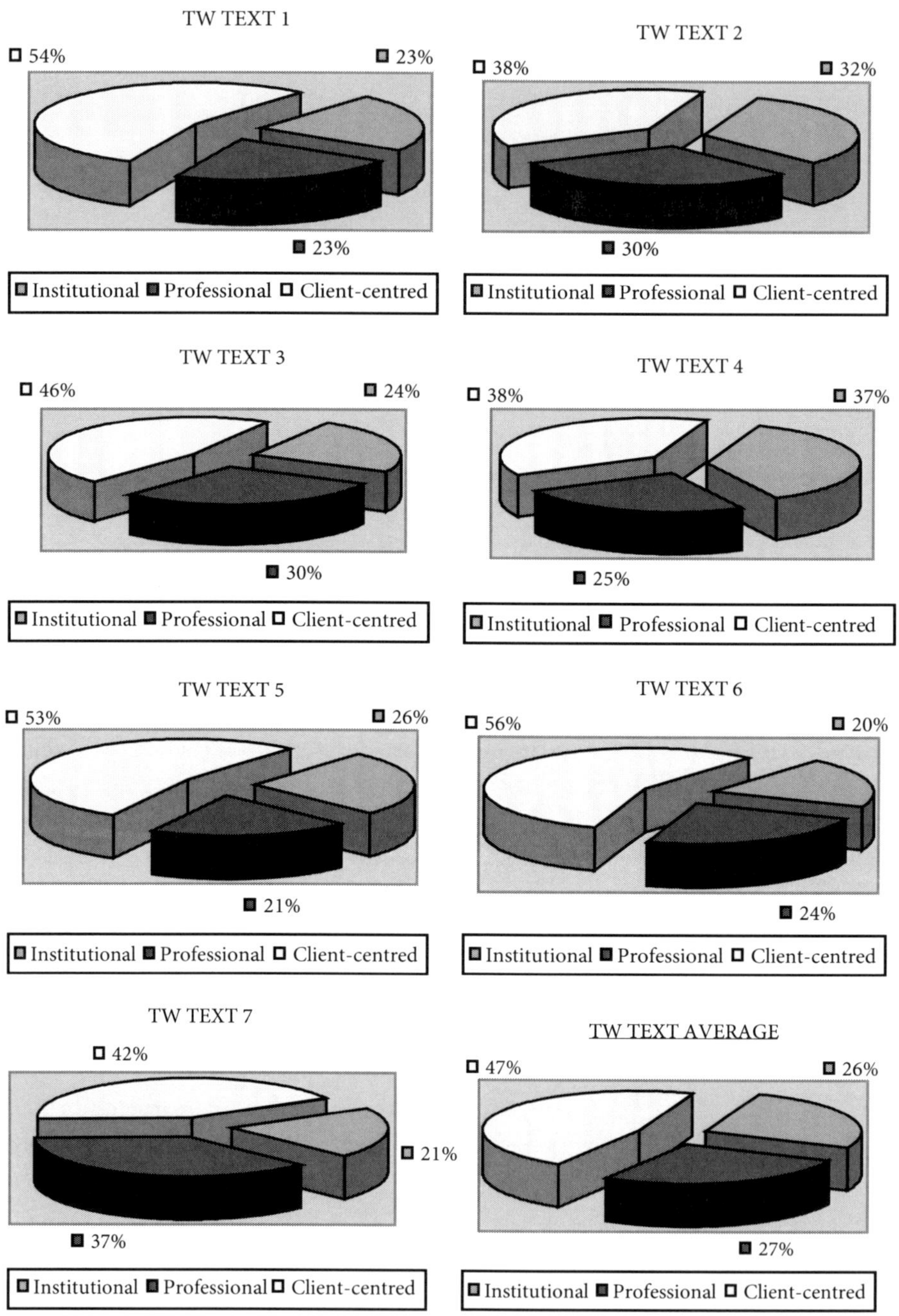
TW TEXT 1
54%
23%
23%
Institutional Professional Client-centred
TW TEXT 2
38%
32%
30%
Institutional Professional Client-centred
TW TEXT 3
46%
24%
30%
Institutional Professional Client-centred
TW TEXT 4
38%
37%
25%
Institutional Professional Client-centred
TW TEXT 5
53%
26%
21%
Institutional Professional Client-centred
TW TEXT 6
56%
20%
24%
Institutional Professional Client-centred
TW TEXT 7
42%
21%
37%
Institutional Professional Client-centred
TW TEXT AVERAGE
47%
26%
27%
Institutional Professional Client-centred

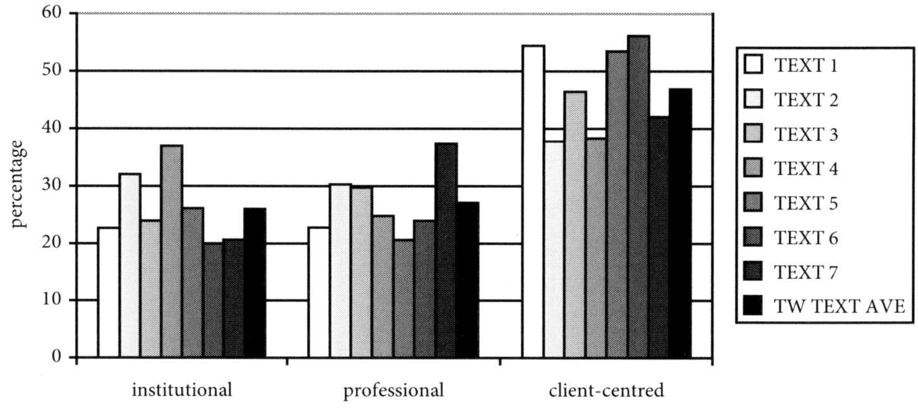

Figure 4.21 Discursive content of TW psychoeducational texts

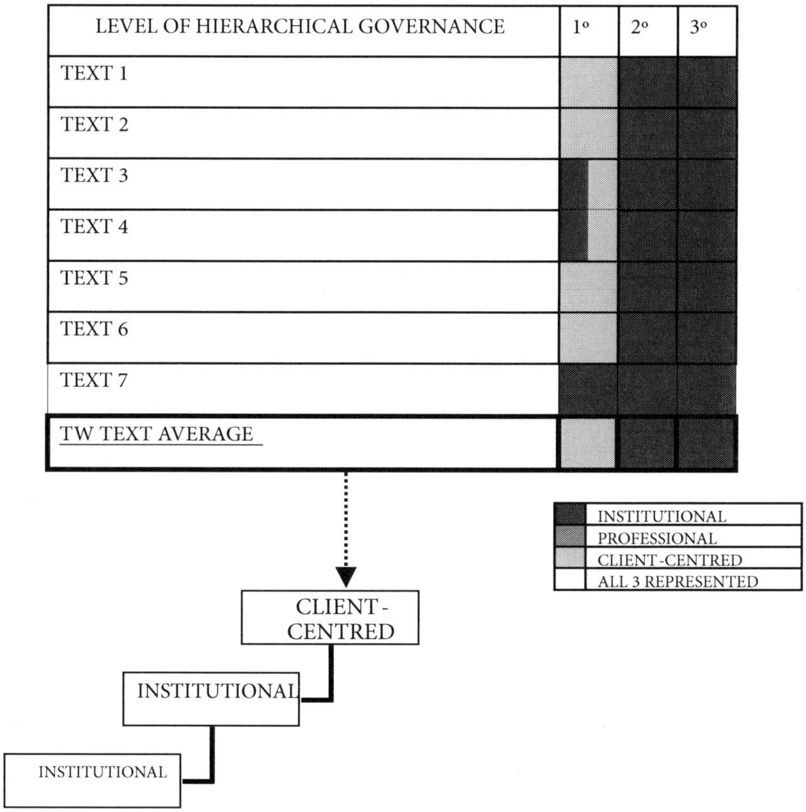

Figure 4.22 Discursive hierarchies of TW psychoeducational texts

at their primary levels reminiscent of the northern PRC texts – the text which addresses schizophrenia conspicuous in this regard – but no variation was found at penultimate levels of the discursive hierarchy: all texts are exclusively institutional in form regardless of topic or content type.

In sum, analysis of the TW psychoeducational texts has revealed a literature that is similar in many respects to that sourced in the PRC, typically presenting as client-centred, although institutional forms are evident. On average, the greater proportion of the texts' discursive content is client-centred, especially the case in texts dealing with clinical depression. Where schizophrenia is addressed as an issue, however, the professional voice of medicine resonates within an institutional discursive presentation.

Analytic findings for the Australian Chinese-language psychoeducational literature

The corpus of Australian (AUS) Chinese-language psychoeducational literature analysed in this study constitutes a body of literature collected in Australia over a period covering 2001–2004. Texts were obtained from the Queensland Transcultural Mental Health Centre, a government-funded specialist mental health service for people of non-English-speaking background living in Queensland, Australia, as well as from the Multicultural Mental Health Australia (MMHA) website (see http://www.mmha.org.au). MMHA is a national association that "links a wide range of state and territory mental health specialists and services, advocacy groups and tertiary institutions to promote the mental health and well being of Australia's diverse communities" (Multicultural Mental Health Australia 2004). Predictably, as a 'minority' language psychoeducational resource, the number of Chinese-language texts available in Australia was more limited compared to the numbers available in the PRC and Taiwan, and there was duplication of texts across the sites of collection. By and large the texts were also shorter in length than their PRC and Taiwanese counterparts. As a consequence, after excluding duplicate texts, the paramount body of texts collected constituted the actual study corpus.

The topics of the eight Australian texts studied cover a similar range as the PRC and Taiwanese corpora – mental illness generically, depression, schizophrenia and caregiving – but unlike the other corpora no single topic dominated. The Australian texts came in the form of A4 infosheets, multi-page pamphlets and a leaflet. Details of the texts are provided in Figure 4.23.

The relative frequencies of rhetorical relations for each of these texts and the average for all AUS texts analysed are presented in Figure 4.24. On aver-

	TEXT 1	TEXT 2	TEXT 3	TEXT 4
Title	怎樣應付家人的精神病 (Coping with mental illness in the family)	甚麼是精神疾病？ (What is mental illness?)	抑鬱症並不是時常真的‘黑與白’: 有關抑鬱症的一些常識 (Depression is never really ‘black and white’: some facts about depression)	精神失常 (Schizophrenia)
Author / publisher	Queensland Transcultural Mental Health Centre	Queensland Transcultural Mental Health Centre	Queensland Transcultural Mental Health Centre	New South Wales Transcultural Mental Health Centre and Westmead Children's Hospital
Year of publication	1999	1999	1999	1999
Place of publication	Brisbane, Australia.	Brisbane, Australia.	Brisbane, Australia.	Sydney, Australia.
Description	2 page plain paper infosheet	3 page plain paper infosheet	3 page plain paper infosheet	6 page plain paper pamphlet
Topic	Mental illness – caregiving	Mental illness – general	Depression	Schizophrenia

	TEXT 5	TEXT 6	TEXT 7	TEXT 8
Title	憂鬱 (Depression)	精神分裂症與年青人 (Schizophrenia and young people)	什麼是精神健康 (What is mental health?)	Caring for carers – Chinese
Author / publisher	New South Wales Transcultural Mental Health Centre and Westmead Children's Hospital	New South Wales Department of Health, NSW Multicultural Health Communication Service	New South Wales Transcultural Mental Health Centre and Westmead Children's Hospital	Australian Transcultural Mental Health Network
Year of publication	1999	1996	1999	c1999
Place of publication	Sydney, Australia.	Sydney, Australia.	Sydney, Australia.	n/a
Description	6 page plain paper pamphlet	4 page plain paper pamphlet	6 page plain paper pamphlet	1 page plain paper leaflet
Topic	Depression	Schizophrenia	Mental illness – general	Mental illness – caregiving

Figure 4.23 Identification details of AUS psychoeducational texts

age, evidence (10.5%) and elaboration (10.4%) comprise the larger proportions of the analysed AUS psychoeducational literature. This stands in distinction to the PRC and TW texts where elaboration alone comprises the larger proportion (16.7% & 26.7%, respectively). Also distinctive to the AUS literature is the very low representation of sequence relations (0.1%) on average compared to the PRC and TW texts (9.6% & 5.5%, respectively) and the higher level of enablement relations (5.6% compared to 0.6% & 1.6%, respectively). Contrast relations on average have a higher representation in the AUS texts than the PRC and TW texts (7.4% compared to 3.5% & 2.2%, respectively), while antithesis relations are lower (1.7% compared to 4.0% & 4.5%, respectively). The significance of this will be taken up in Chapter 5, simply to note here that antithesis and contrast are 'fraternal' relations: contrast entailing a balanced, non-value-laden comparison; antithesis, a positioned, value-laden comparison underpinned by incompatibility.

Distinctive in relation to text topics in the AUS corpus is the higher than average level of enablement relations (10.6% & 19.0%, respectively) obtained in Text 1 and Text 8, both dealing with the issue of caring for people with a mental illness. A higher than average level of enablement relations also occurs in the TW text dealing with caregiving. Enablement makes possible the performing of an action by the reader.

Like the PRC and TW corpora, restatement, summary and justification relations are minimally represented in the AUS psychoeducational literature, both on average and within individual texts.

Relations	TEXT 1		TEXT 2		TEXT 3		TEXT 4		TEXT 5	
	nos	%(rnd)	nos	%(rnd)	nos	%(rnd)	nos	%(rnd)	nos	%(rnd)
ant	2	3	1	0.9	0	0	0	0	0	0
bgd	2	3	0	0	2	2.3	0	0	2	2.3
ccl	1	1.5	0	0	0	0	2	2.7	0	0
ccn	5	7.6	1	0.9	3	3.4	4	5.4	2	2.3
cdn	7	10.6	7	6.1	4	4.5	3	4.1	1	1.1
cir	1	1.5	4	3.5	8	9.1	6	8.1	9	10.3
cnt	5	7.6	6	5.3	6	6.8	6	8.1	6	6.9
elb	6	9.1	12	10.5	12	13.6	8	10.8	14	16.1
enb	7	10.6	5	4.4	6	6.8	0	0	0	0
evd	9	13.6	8	7	11	12.5	10	13.5	11	12.6
evl	2	3	4	3.5	1	1.1	3	4.1	3	3.4
jt	5	7.6	16	14	7	8	7	9.5	11	12.6
jus	0	0	0	0	0	0	0	0	0	0

lst	0	0	12	10.5	6	6.8	3	4.1	3	3.4
mns	0	0	1	0.9	1	1.1	0	0	1	1.1
mot	4	6.1	11	9.6	1	1.1	1	1.4	1	1.1
pur	1	1.5	4	3.5	1	1.1	3	4.1	2	2.3
rea	4	6.1	1	0.9	1	1.1	2	2.7	2	2.3
res	1	1.5	9	7.9	9	10.2	10	13.5	11	12.6
rtt	0	0	1	0.9	0	0	0	0	0	0
seq	0	0	0	0	0	0	0	0	1	1.1
sol	4	6.1	11	9.6	9	10.2	6	8.1	7	8
sum	0	0	0	0	0	0	0	0	0	0
TOTAL	66	100	114	100	88	100	74	100	87	100

Relations	TEXT 6		TEXT 7		TEXT 8		AUS Text Average
	nos	%(rnd)	nos	%(rnd)	nos	%(rnd)	%(rnd)
ant	1	2	2	2.8	1	4.8	1.7
bgd	1	2	0	0	0	0	1.2
ccl	1	2	0	0	1	4.8	1.4
ccn	3	6.1	2	2.8	0	0	3.6
cdn	4	8.2	2	2.8	1	4.8	5.3
cir	2	4.1	7	9.7	2	9.5	7
cnt	4	8.2	8	11.1	1	4.8	7.4
elb	4	8.2	4	5.6	2	9.5	10.4
enb	2	4.1	0	0	4	19	5.6
evd	2	4.1	15	20.8	0	0	10.5
evl	2	4.1	2	2.8	1	4.8	3.4
jt	4	8.2	4	5.6	1	4.8	8.8
jus	0	0	0	0	0	0	0
lst	0	0	2	2.8	0	0	3.5
mns	0	0	0	0	0	0	0.4
mot	3	6.1	1	1.4	3	14.3	5.1
pur	0	0	3	4.2	2	9.5	3.3
rea	8	16.3	2	2.8	0	0	4
res	6	12.2	11	15.3	1	4.8	9.8
rtt	0	0	0	0	0	0	0.1
seq	0	0	0	0	0	0	0.1
sol	2	4.1	7	9.7	1	4.8	7.6
sum	0	0	0	0	0	0	0
TOTAL	49	100	72	100	21	100	100

Figure 4.24 Relative frequencies in AUS psychoeducational texts

Figure 4.25 illustrates the proportional discursive content of each text as well as the average for all AUS texts analysed. In contrast to the other corpora, on average, professional discourse represents proportionally the largest discursive presence, eclipsing the client-centred and the institutional, although not constituting a majority (> 50%). While four of the texts (Texts 1, 4, 6 & 7) individually follow this discursive pattern, client-centredness is proportionally largest in three texts (Texts 3, 5 & 8) and institutional discourse proportionally largest in the other (Text 2). Two of the client-centred exceptions (Texts 3 & 5) comprise the AUS texts addressing clinical depression. Well above average levels of client-centredness are also characteristic of the TW texts dealing with depression. Nevertheless, here client-centredness is *not* mediated by sequence relations (narrative).

The other disease-specific texts (Texts 4 & 6), dealing with schizophrenia, have below average levels of client-centredness (30% & 29%, respectively), strongly resonating the professional voice of medicine (45% & 47%, respectively). Well above average levels of professional discourse are a feature of texts from the other corpora which address schizophrenia and related psychoses.

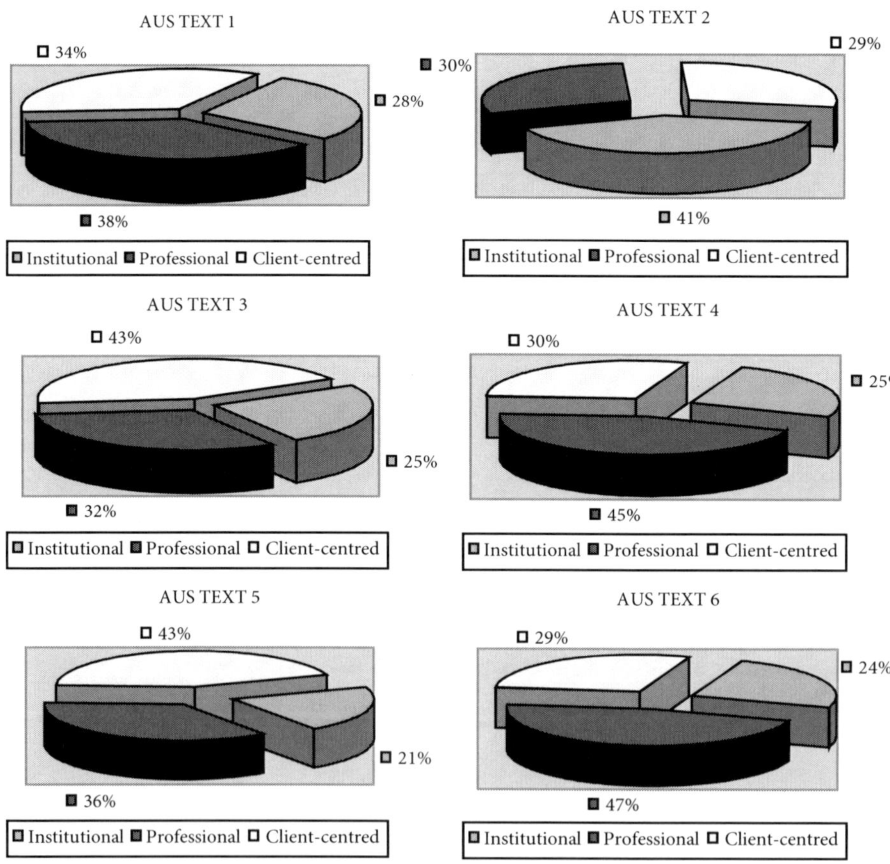

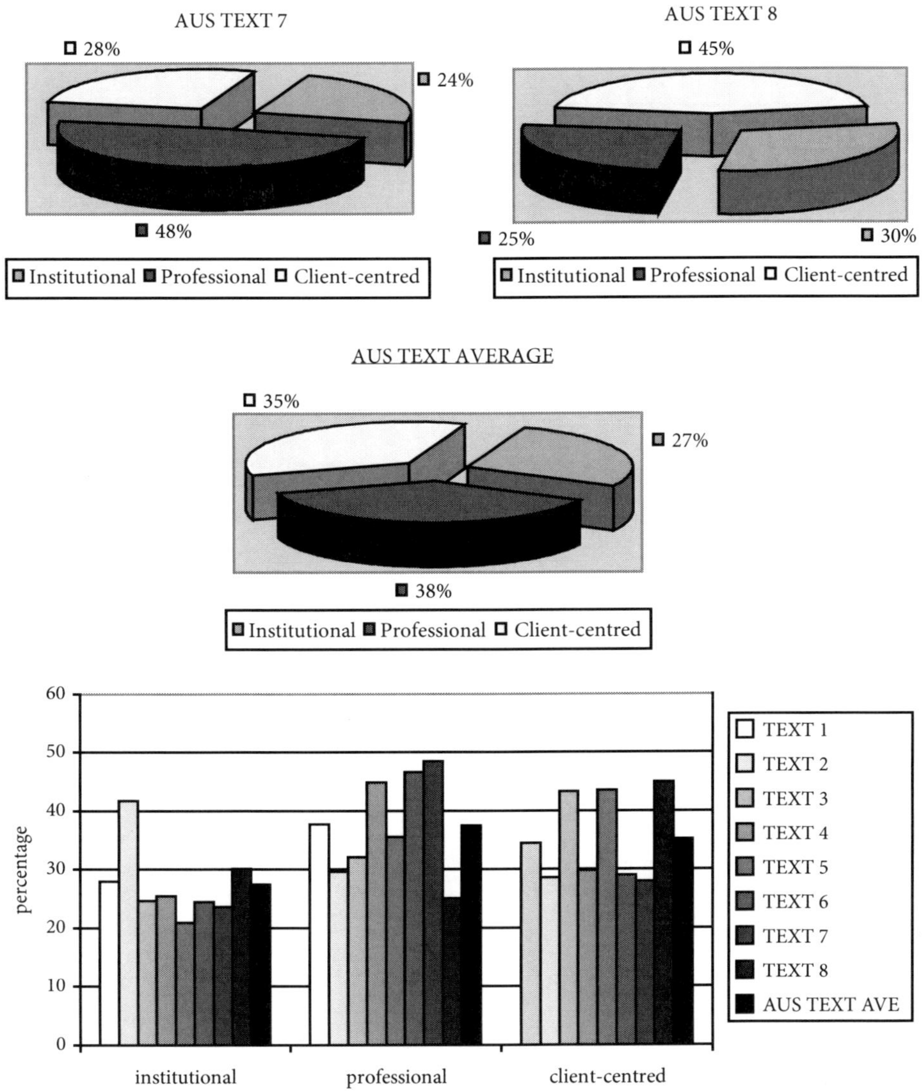

Figure 4.25 Discursive content of AUS psychoeducational texts

Figure 4.26 illustrates the discursive hierarchies of the AUS psychoeducational texts and the AUS text average. In contrast to the other corpora, client-centredness no longer dominates the highest level of the discursive hierarchy. Here, institutional and professional discursive forms are now more highly evident, with client-centredness 'slipping back' to the penultimate levels of discursive governance and beyond. In nearly all AUS texts, the institutional voice governs penultimate levels.

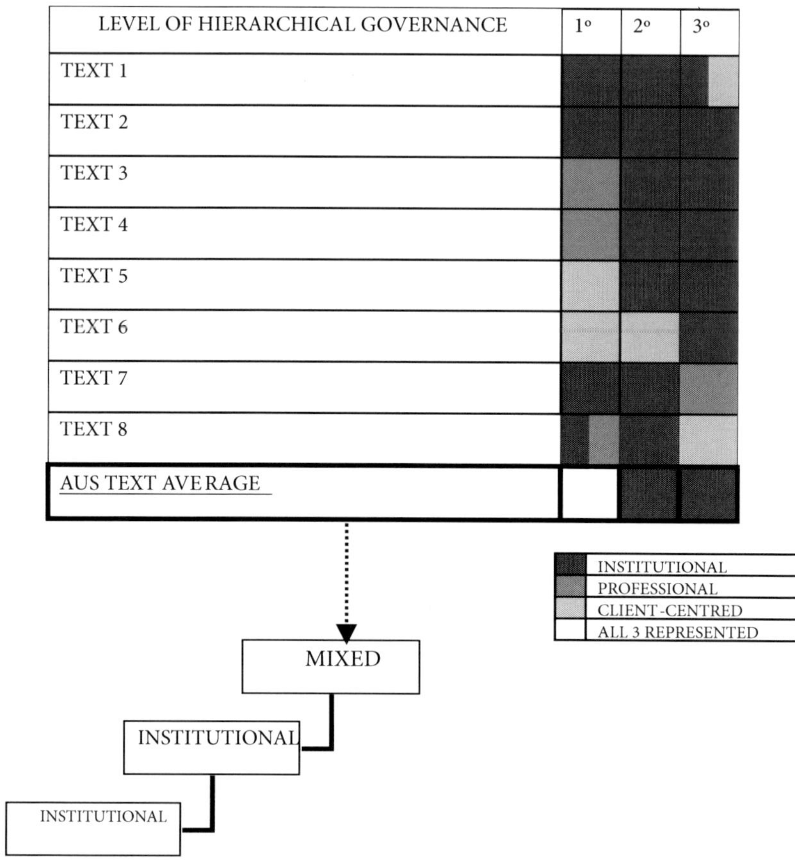

Figure 4.26 Discursive hierarchies of AUS psychoeducational texts

Unlike the AUS texts dealing generically with mental illness or the issue of caregiving, those dealing with specific illnesses (schizophrenia and clinical depression) are dominated by client-centredness or the professional voice of medicine at their highest level of discursive governance. However, there is no consistency within these topic groups at this level. As pointed out above, the penultimate levels of these texts are predominantly institutional in character. Further exploration of this relationship between topic and discursive form follows in Chapter 5.

In sum, analysis of the AUS Chinese-language psychoeducational texts has revealed a literature that for the most part presents as institutionalised, with client-centred forms present but less dominant than in PRC and TW literature. On average, the greater proportion of the AUS texts' discursive content resonates the professional voice of medicine, in stark contrast to the other corpora. This is especially the case for texts dealing with schizophrenia.

The discursive form of Chinese-language psychoeducational literature

The chapter has explicated the discursive form of the texts under study using the RST analytic framework. RST has proved to be an effective tool for this, allowing explication of discursive content *and* hierarchy. The chapter has identified a number of similarities and differences within and across the PRC, TW and AUS corpora. In terms of Fairclough's model of discourse analysis presented in the previous chapter, the interpositioning of text and discursive practice has been examined so far. In so doing, the first two questions pertaining to discourse analysis of 'multivocal' text, as raised in Chapter 3, have been addressed, namely, Question One: What characterises the different voices of the text? (see in particular Figure 4.10); and Question Two: When does each voice speak? (see in particular Figures 4.16, 4.17, 4.18, 4.21, 4.22, 4.25 & 4.26).

In the next chapter, comparisons across psychoeducational corpora will be undertaken and the potential communicative efficacy of the literature under study will be evaluated in light of these comparative findings.

CHAPTER 5

Shaping minds

The introductory chapter of this volume drew attention to the desirability of society at large and people with a mental illness and their carers ascribing appropriate meaning to mental illness, that is, embracing a conceptual explanatory model that is in harmony with cultural beliefs yet, at the same time, overcomes the stigma and prejudices fixed in tradition. It was noted that the explanatory model employed by health professionals in the West at present, and for the most part across the globe, is founded on a highly biomedicalised conception of mental illness. This conception views imbalances in the body's neurochemistry as the aetiological basis for mental illness, and promotes the timely use of medication and adjunct therapies as the key to alleviation of clinical signs. Such an explanatory model of mental illness is utilised in the West in government public health campaigns to educate the broader community about mental illness. In so doing, health care bodies hope that the lives of people with a mental illness and their carers are improved by shaping a constructive and sympathetic understanding of mental illness within the minds of the broader population. At the same time, as discussed in Chapter 3 of this volume, shaping minds in such a way positions the health care provider at the centre of the community's (and the family's and the individual's) response to mental illness, replicating institutionally-derived power inequalities already deeply entrenched in most societies. This has led to calls for a more client-centred approach to mental illness and mental health care: one which places greater emphasis on life experience and empowerment of the health consumer, with lesser emphasis placed on the essential role of medicine, health professional and health institution.

The introductory chapter also brought to light the importance of consideration of culture in achieving effective community psychoeducation. In Chapter 2, the prevailing lay conception of mental illness in contemporary Chinese societies was shown to be heterogenous, encompassing traditional ancestral, spiritual, mystical, somatic and genetic aetiologies, alongside the biomedical model propagated by Western medicine. A plurality of understandings pertaining to disease pathogenesis, appropriate pathways to care and the proper treatment of mental illness was found to characterise Chinese populations across the diaspora. Chapter 2 also noted that the biomedical conception of mental illness dominates health professional understandings in China and Taiwan. This accords with the proposition presented in Chapter 1 that Western biomedicine would likely inform the prevailing explanatory model of health and illness amongst public health professionals across the developed and the developing world. Chapter 2, however, cautioned that such a conception coincides with traditional stigmatic notions of mental illness based on heredity at the same time as legitimising the eugenic vision that maintains currency in mainland China today.

Drawing on the results of the analysis undertaken in Chapter 4, the current chapter explores how the biomedical explanatory model of mental illness embraced by health professionals across the Chinese diaspora is communicated in the community psychoeducational literature under study. The chapter examines how the psychoeducational message is discursively represented and how this representation intersects with the salient cultural understandings documented in Chapter 2. Similarities and differences in the discursive form of the literature sourced from the three sites under study are discussed and considered in terms of their potential influence on effective communication of the intended psychoeducational message. Reasons for differential formulation of the psychoeducational message across the Chinese diaspora (mainland China, Taiwan and Australia) are contemplated.

Shaping minds in mainland Chinese and Taiwanese psychoeducational literature

In promulgating a professional explanatory model of mental illness grounded in the biomedical conception, Chapter 4 reveals a mainland Chinese and Taiwanese psychoeducational literature distinguished by substantial resonance of the client-centred voice, both in terms of discursive proportion as well as hierarchy. Although the professional explanatory model of mental illness in mainland China and Taiwan, like that in the West, is informed by biomedicine, mainland Chinese and Taiwanese psychoeducational texts are not distinguished discursively by greater resonance of the professional voice of medicine. This finding suggests a preferred communicative form for the representation of mental illness in mainland Chinese and Taiwanese community psychoeducational literature. This preferred form places significant value on client-centred representations. The results of Chapter 4 indicate that client-centredness here is overwhelmingly characterised by the voice of the lifeworld, mediated by narrative and the provision of detail, and rarely extends to empowerment and active choice.

This use of the voice of the lifeworld as a discursive strategy has precedence in mainland China, where it is commonplace in news text. It is not unusual to encounter extensive narrative in mainland Chinese news bulletins, print stories and political genre in order to draw attention to an issue of concern (Lu 2000;

Qiu 2000; Wang 2002). The power of narrative in persuasive communication, of course, has been recognised across many cultural settings, storytelling being "one of the oldest and most quintessential human of activities" (Gwyn 2002, p. 139). Narrative's persuasive potential emerges from its ability "to impart a vision of reality and one that is at once socially positioned and culturally grounded", which sees narrative serve as an effective cultural conduit for the dissemination of messages, particularly in indigenous settings (Garro & Mattingly 2000b, p. 260). Lu (2000, p. 7), in fact, documents a narrative tradition in Chinese rhetoric, where anecdotes comprise part of a discursive armoury employed by Chinese writers "as means of persuasion for the purpose of moral teaching, political control and expediency, and interpersonal manipulation." Despite the passing of ages, in contemporary Chinese writings such devices, Lu (2000, p. 7) states,

> remain fundamentally the same. Even in contemporary Chinese rhetoric and communication, we see classical themes and forms resurface, sometimes being appropriated or displaced for various purposes. Such phenomena indicate the enduring force of Chinese rhetorical culture and the relationship between rhetoric and culture.

Recent movement toward consumer interests in the West has seen greater use of narrative in persuasive communication here, for example, in advertising. Its broader potential in health communication also has been acknowledged, given that

> hearing narrative accounts is a principle means through which cultural understandings about illness – including possible causes, appropriate social responses, healing strategies, and characteristics of therapeutic alternatives – are acquired, confirmed, refined or modified. (Garro & Mattingly 2000a, p. 26)

Chapter 4 of this volume, however, has found that while narrative clearly features in indigenous Chinese psychoeducational literature and is a key contributor to the client-centredness that ultimately differentiates the indigenous Chinese literature, this is not the case for Australian psychoeducational literature targeting Chinese-speaking migrants. Here, narrative is rarely encountered despite recognition of its value in persuasive communication, particularly health communication.

Chapter 4 has also found that client-centredness in indigenous Chinese psychoeducational literature is rarely characterised by empowerment and active choice, in contrast to the Australian psychoeducational literature. This limited expression of empowerment in the indigenous Chinese psychoeducational literature accords with Confucian notions of direction by authority and collective responsibility. Such values subordinate concern for the individual and valorise respect for and compliance to those in positions of power and in possession of specialised knowledge (Fan & Karnilowicz 2000; Kung 2001). Kleinman (1980,

p. 264) has observed that in Chinese societies the health practitioner's "secret knowledge, somewhat higher social status, and emotional distance are signs of his therapeutic power and, therefore, are an essential part of the doctor-patient relationship." Accordingly, the cultural expectation in relation to the psychoeducational message would be instruction by the authority (here, public health body) as to the appropriate course of action and how to accomplish it (Pearson 1995c). This appears to manifest in the literature under study through silencing of consumer empowerment and resonance of the institutional voice.

The client-centredness distinguishing the indigenous Chinese psychoeducational literature results in a discursive understating of the professional voice of medicine. This accords, as raised in Chapter 2, with the fact that a biomedical conception of mental illness may legitimise the biogenetic component to cultural stigma salient to Chinese societies, which views mental illness as running in family lines. Privileging of the biomedical agenda in community psychoeducation, therefore, could be counterproductive by serving to reinforce the very cultural phenomenon that psychoeducation seeks to overcome. The study's findings for the mainland Chinese and Taiwanese psychoeducational corpora, therefore, point to a notably client-centred literature that understates the professional voice of medicine, seemingly reflecting normative persuasive communication in Chinese culture and the potential intersection of the biomedical conception of mental illness with Chinese cultural stigma.

Shaping minds in Australian Chinese-language psychoeducational literature

The Australian corpus is distinct from the other two under study in that it comprises text produced for Chinese communities where they are a minority population-wise, albeit one of the largest migrant populations in Australia. Here, as described in Chapter 2 of this volume, Chinese cultural explanatory models of mental illness and culture-bound stigma differ from those of Anglo-dominant Australian society. In the introductory chapter it was noted that, in order to produce effective psychoeducation in the target community, culture needs to be taken into account. However, an ever-present danger in the migrant setting is that messages formulated by public health bodies, while effective for achieving belief change in dominant society, may not be effective for changing beliefs prevailing in minority co-cultures. Thus, if discursive strategies developed for dominant society psychoeducation 'colonise' minority group psychoeducational texts, a loss in communicative efficacy may result.

The results of Chapter 4 suggest that colonisation is evident in the Australian Chinese-language psychoeducational literature. On average, the Australian Chinese-language psychoeducational literature substantially resonates the professional voice of medicine, notably more so than the indigenous Chinese texts. Compared to the indigenous Chinese texts, the professional voice of medicine is more resonant proportionally and fields a greater presence in the higher levels of discursive governance. Given the deemed effectiveness of biomedicalising mental illness as a community psychoeducational strategy in the West, these findings from Chapter 4 suggest a colonisation of psychoeducational literature targeting Chinese-speaking migrants residing in Australia by discursive phenomena characterising Anglo-dominant society. Put simply, what has been deemed effective for bringing about belief change in dominant society has been replicated when seeking to bring about belief change in minority co-cultures.

The hegemony of dominant society discursive strategies is further confirmed by the lack of uniformity across individual texts comprising the Australian corpus as compared to the indigenous Chinese corpora. Despite the professional voice of medicine resonating proportionally largest in the typical Australian text, the client-centred voice resonates largest in three individual Australian texts and the institutional voice in one text (see Figure 4.25, this volume). What is more, all three discursive voices dominate the primary level of discursive governance across individual Australian texts (see Figure 4.26). This discursive profile of the Australian corpus is distinct from that of the indigenous Chinese corpora, where individual texts for the most part mirror corpus averages in terms of trend and where variation across individual texts, when it occurs, can be accounted for by disease topic. Variation evident in all corpora arising from disease topic is discussed subsequently.

Chapter 3 of this volume noted the contemporary debate in the West over preferred representations of mental illness. An alternative client-centred explanatory model of mental illness, one which promotes life experience and consumer empowerment, has emerged of late to challenge the biomedical conception that has come to dominate the health profession and lay society alike in the West. This dominant society debate manifests in the Australian psychoeducational literature targeting Chinese-speaking migrants, with some Australian Chinese-language texts strongly resonating the professional voice of medicine while others strongly resonate the client-centred voice. Once again, a hegemony of discursive phenomena salient to dominant society is evident in texts targeting minority co-cultures. Dominant society debate over preferred conceptions of mental illness and approaches to mental health care, namely biomedical versus client-centred, which sees one or the other propagated or, at least, accommodated by public health bodies, hegemonicly resonates in psychoeducational literature intended for Chinese-speaking migrants.

Ironically, the hegemony of competing discourses at first glance sees some of the Australian Chinese-language psychoeducational texts, namely those that resonate the client-centred voice, field discursive forms similar to those that characterise the indigenous Chinese texts. However, unlike the indigenous Chinese texts, client-centredness in the Australian literature is mediated by sizable quantities of enablement (AUS text average = 5.6%) and contrast relations (AUS text average = 7.4%). The combined frequencies of enablement and contrast relations is equal to or exceeds the frequency of elaboration relations in five of the eight Australian texts under study (AUS texts 1, 3, 6, 7 & 8), often exceeding by large amounts. Moreover, the frequency of enablement relations alone exceeds that of elaboration relations in two of these Australian texts (Texts 1 & 8) and the frequency of contrast relations is on par with or exceeds that of elaboration relations in another two texts (Texts 6 & 7).

Such a finding is unprecedented in the indigenous Chinese texts, where enablement and contrast relations are of minimal significance (in combination or taken individually) when compared to the dominant relation mediating client-centredness in the indigenous Chinese texts (elaboration or sequence). Figure 5.1 illustrates this difference in the mediation of client-centredness across Australian and indigenous Chinese corpora. Narrative (sequence) features in the latter but is virtually absent from the former. The converse applies for enablement relations, which mediate empowerment. Contrast relations, which also mediate empowerment through the expression of active choice, also field higher frequency in the Australian corpus as compared to the indigenous Chinese corpora. Figure 5.1 further shows that mediation of option or alternative differs across these corpora. While the frequency of contrast relations, where a balanced comparison of options is proffered without indication of preference, is higher in the Australian corpus, the frequency of antithesis relations, where an incompatibility deemed to exist between options commands a preferred option, is higher in the indigenous Chinese corpora. Simply put, contrast allows one relative freedom to follow one course of action or another, while antithesis obliges one to follow one course of action at the expense of another. This study's data, therefore, indicates that the expression of options and alternatives in the indigenous Chinese corpus is more contained than that in the Australian corpus, with the former resorting more to the authoritative imperative and the latter facilitating active choice.

This discursive profile indicates that empowerment and the provision of choice are salient features of the Australian corpus. This is not the case for the indigenous Chinese corpora. Such a profile likely reflects dominant societal notions

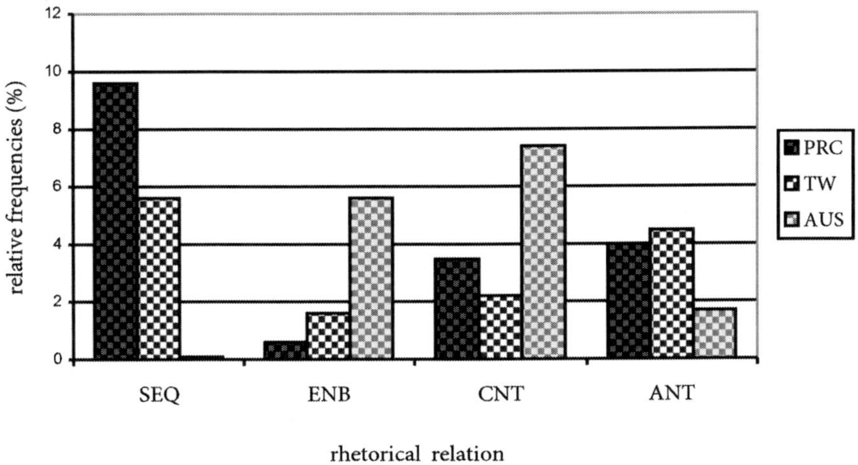

Figure 5.1 Client-centredness mediated in PRC, TW and AUS psychoeducational texts: comparison of sequence/enablement/contrast/antithesis relative frequencies

of importance of the individual in Australia, which appear to have colonised public health literature targeting a minority migrant group. In light of the valorisation of Confucian notions of direction by authority and compliant response in Chinese culture, as reported in Chapter 2 of this volume, the colonisation of texts targeting Chinese-speaking migrants by antithetical notions of empowerment and choice in the end may prove problematic for the target readership and consequently lower the communicative efficacy of the texts concerned.

Shaping minds across the Chinese diaspora

This section continues the comparative discussion by foregrounding the similarities and differences in the discursive form of the literature sourced from the three sites under study and evaluating their potential influence on effective communication of the intended psychoeducational message. In the previous section, differences in the resonance of the professional voice of medicine across Australian and indigenous Chinese corpora were highlighted and explained in terms of dominant society discursive hegemony. Differences in the resonance of the professional voice of medicine across corpora *and* across individual texts comprising the corpora are explored below.

Figure 5.2 reaffirms that the Australian Chinese-language psychoeducational literature, on average, more strongly resonates the professional voice of medicine

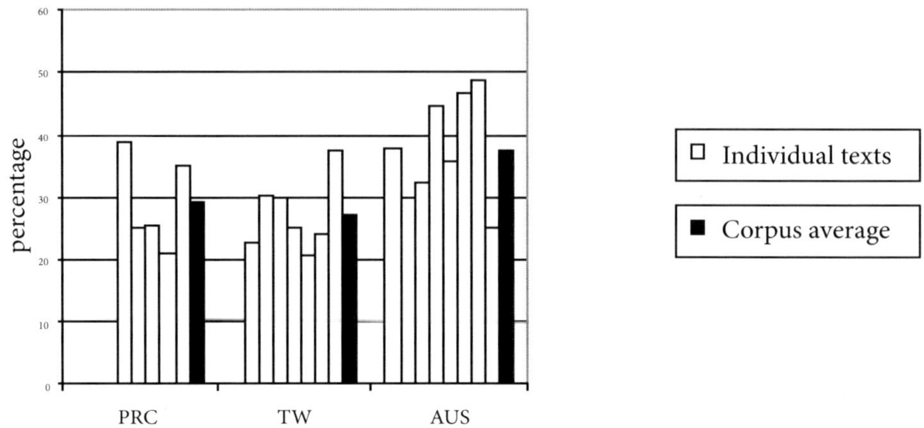

Figure 5.2 Comparison of professional discursive content across PRC, TW and AUS psychoeducational texts

than its indigenous Chinese counterparts.[1] From the perspective of individual texts, only one of the Australian texts under study possesses a level of professional discourse (slightly) below the mainland Chinese and Taiwanese averages. It already has been noted in this volume that a psychoeducational message intended for Chinese communities which overstates the biomedical explanatory model of mental illness in the end may be counterproductive. Kung (2001, pp. 98–99), for example, observes "cases in which siblings of [Chinese] patients became very disturbed over the psychiatrists' remark on a genetic factor as the cause of mental disorder." This has clear ramifications for the communicative efficacy of the Australian psychoeducational corpus given its higher resonance of the professional voice of medicine when compared to the indigenous Chinese corpora. Any overstating of the biomedical message may intersect with cultural stigma based on heredity, merely augmenting the cultural beliefs that the psychoeducational message intends to overcome.

Figure 5.2 also shows that individual indigenous Chinese texts do possess levels of professional discourse approaching the Australian corpus average. Disease topic provides some explanation for this phenomenon. Chapter 4 of this volume documented higher than corpus-average proportions of professional discourse in individual psychoeducational texts that specifically addressed schizophrenia and

1. SPSS 16.0 analysis of variance found difference between AUS and PRC corpora approaching significance at $p = 0.060$; difference between AUS and TW corpora significant at $p = 0.014$; and no significant difference between PRC and TW corpora ($p = 0.645$).

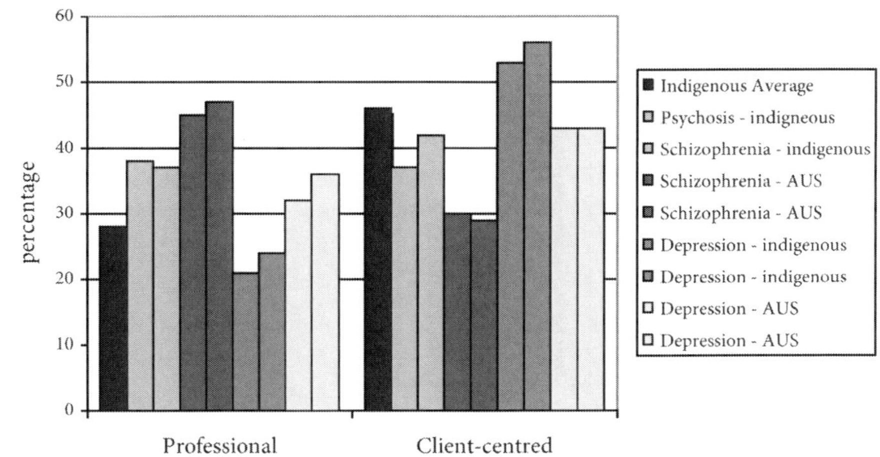

Figure 5.3 Comparison of professional and client-centred discursive content across indigenous Chinese[2] and AUS corpora according to disease topic

related psychoses. This occurred across all corpora. It appears that greater resonance of the professional voice of medicine characterises texts dealing with a disease whose 'positive' symptoms such as delusions and hallucinations particularly challenge societal norms of behaviour. There appears to be greater resorting to the professional voice where the disease experience is exceptionally confronting and social stigma especially intense. Even in indigenous Chinese psychoeducational texts, where normative persuasive communication and the genetic component to stigma determine a relative understating of the biomedical model, greater voicing of this model occurs when addressing schizophrenia and psychosis.

Figure 5.3 shows that Australian and indigenous Chinese texts dealing with schizophrenia and psychosis possess levels of professional discourse higher than the average level found in the indigenous Chinese corpora. Levels in the Australian texts are particularly high given the higher base-line level found in the Australian corpus as compared to the indigenous Chinese corpora. It appears that where the biomedical explanatory model of mental illness is broadly accepted by dominant society or, at least, remains culturally unproblematic (Australia), and where schizophrenia and psychosis are the topics of concern, the professional voice of medicine resonates loudest. An Australian psychoeducational message of

2. Given the parity in average values obtained for the indigenous Chinese corpora (professional = 27% & 29%; client-centred = 45% & 47%), combined averages (professional = 28% & client-centred = 46%) form the normative values employed here.

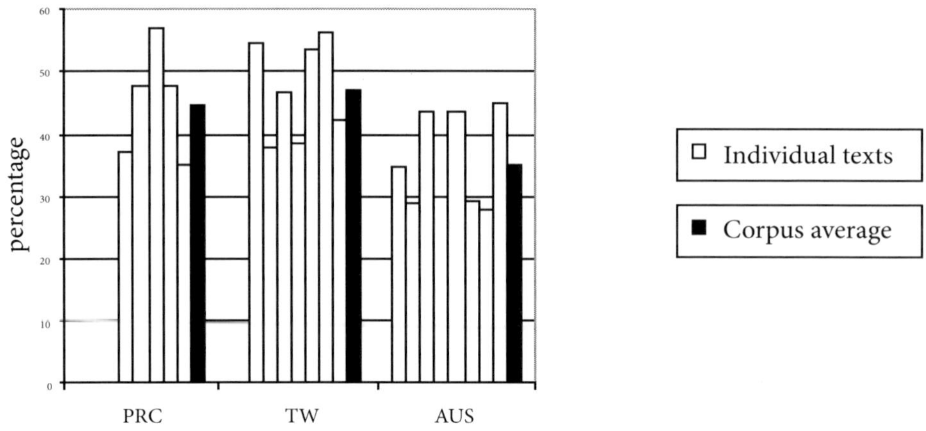

Figure 5.4 Comparison of client-centred discursive content across PRC, TW and AUS psychoeducational texts

this type is likely to be particularly counterproductive when targeting Chinese-speaking migrants, for reasons stated earlier.

The higher levels of professional discourse in psychoeducational texts dealing with schizophrenia and psychosis produce particularly marked below-indigenous-Chinese-average levels of client-centred discourse in the Australian texts (see Figure 5.3). This may bring the communicative efficacy of the Australian literature dealing with schizophrenia further into question, given indigenous Chinese norms for persuasive communication. Levels of client-centredness in the indigenous Chinese texts dealing with schizophrenia and psychosis remain close to average, possibly maintaining levels that meet expectations for normative communication.

A greater resonance of the client-centred voice, on average, in indigenous Chinese psychoeducational literature when compared to Australian literature is reaffirmed in Figure 5.4.[3] As to individual texts, Figure 5.4 shows that all the indigenous Chinese texts analysed possess proportions of client-centred discourse equal to or above the Australian corpus average. Moreover, no Australian texts exceed the mainland Chinese and Taiwanese averages. These findings add weight to the claim made in this study that client-centredness, characterised by the voice of the lifeworld in indigenous Chinese psychoeducational literature, represents a normative form for persuasive communication in Chinese culture.

3. SPSS 16.0 analysis of variance found difference between AUS and PRC corpora significant at $p = 0.049$; difference between AUS and TW corpora significant at $p = 0.011$; and no significant difference between PRC and TW corpora ($p = 0.668$).

Figure 5.4 also shows that individual Australian texts do possess levels of client-centred discourse approaching the indigenous Chinese corpus average. Once again, disease topic provides some explanation for this phenomenon. Chapter 4 of this volume documented higher than corpus-average proportions of client-centred discourse in individual psychoeducational texts that specifically addressed clinical depression. This occurred across all corpora. It appears that greater resonance of the client-centred voice characterises texts dealing with a disease whose symptoms can be interpreted more within the frame of normative social behaviour and experience. Particularly in the case of indigenous Chinese psychoeducational literature, there seems less need to foreground the professional voice of medicine, which risks intersecting with stigmatic conceptions in Chinese culture, where the disease experience is not overtly fear-provoking and strongly stigmatised in society.

Figure 5.3 confirms that indigenous Chinese texts dealing with clinical depression possess higher than average levels of client-centred discourse. Australian texts, typically more biomedicalised than their indigenous Chinese counterparts, also demonstrate greater client-centredness when addressing depression, with levels approaching the indigenous Chinese corpus average. However, client-centredness in the Australian texts, it must be remembered, resonates empowerment and active choice to a much greater extent than indigenous Chinese texts. An Australian psychoeducational message of this type would not accord with the normative expectations of a Chinese-speaking audience anticipating direction and instruction.

Figure 5.3 also confirms that psychoeducational texts addressing clinical depression display much lower resonance of the professional voice of medicine than texts addressing schizophrenia and psychosis. Nevertheless, the Australian depression texts still possess above-indigenous-Chinese-average levels of professional discourse and this relative overstatement of the biomedical message in these texts may prove counter-effective for a Chinese audience, given the biogenetic component to cultural stigma.

As text produced by organisational bodies, it is not surprising that the institutional voice notably resonates in the psychoeducational literature under study (see Chapter 3, this volume). This was confirmed in Chapter 4, with a common institutional 'core' evident in all corpora. The average proportion of institutional discourse is analogous across diasporic sites (see Figure 5.5),[4] in contrast to the variation found in professional and client-centred discourse. There is relative

4. SPSS 16.0 analysis of variance found no significant difference between AUS and PRC corpora ($p = 0.732$); no significant difference between AUS and TW corpora ($p = 0.702$); and no significant difference between PRC and TW corpora ($p = 0.996$).

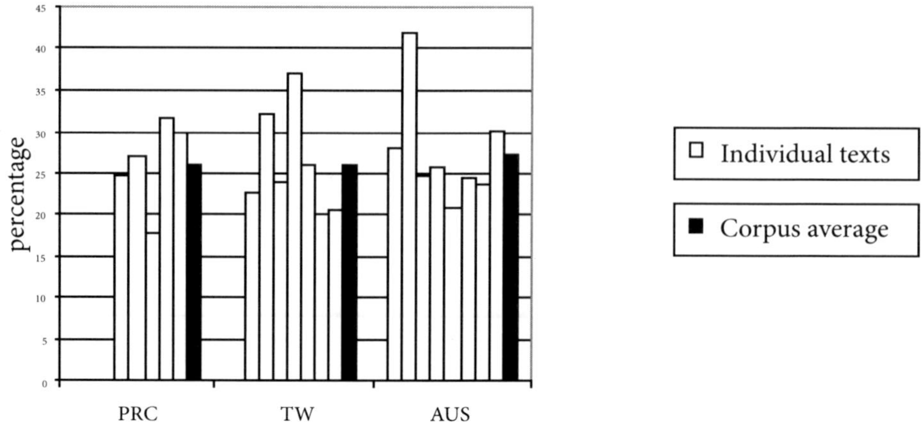

Figure 5.5 Comparison of institutional discursive content across PRC, TW and AUS psychoeducational texts

uniformity across individual texts comprising the corpora, with only one text from each corpus displaying a level of institutionality that diverges markedly from the bulk of the texts under study: the mainland Chinese compilation of narratives about mental illness predictably resonates the lowest level of institutional voice; while a Taiwanese text originating from the United States and one of the Australian texts examining mental illness generically are highly institutional in discursive content. There is no marked preponderance of any single institutional-signifying relation in either of these texts and no demonstrable topic-specific correlation, so it appears that greater resonance of the institutional voice may characterise a minority of psychoeducational texts produced in the West, possibly reflecting a more traditional view of the authoritative position of medicine and health care providers.

The mostly uniform institutionality of the public health literature under study suggests that, in the case of health communication, organisational phenomena appear to transcend political and cultural boundaries. Thus, while the study has determined that approaches to communication of the psychoeducational message vary across indigenous Chinese and Western (migrant) settings in terms of the extent of biomedicalisation and client-centredness and the extent to which client-centredness is expressed through life experience and consumer empowerment, the uniform affirmation of institutional control and authority and the rules and boundaries that sustain this control and authority across the texts under study highlights the unyielding nature of organisational phenomena in institutional communication of this type.

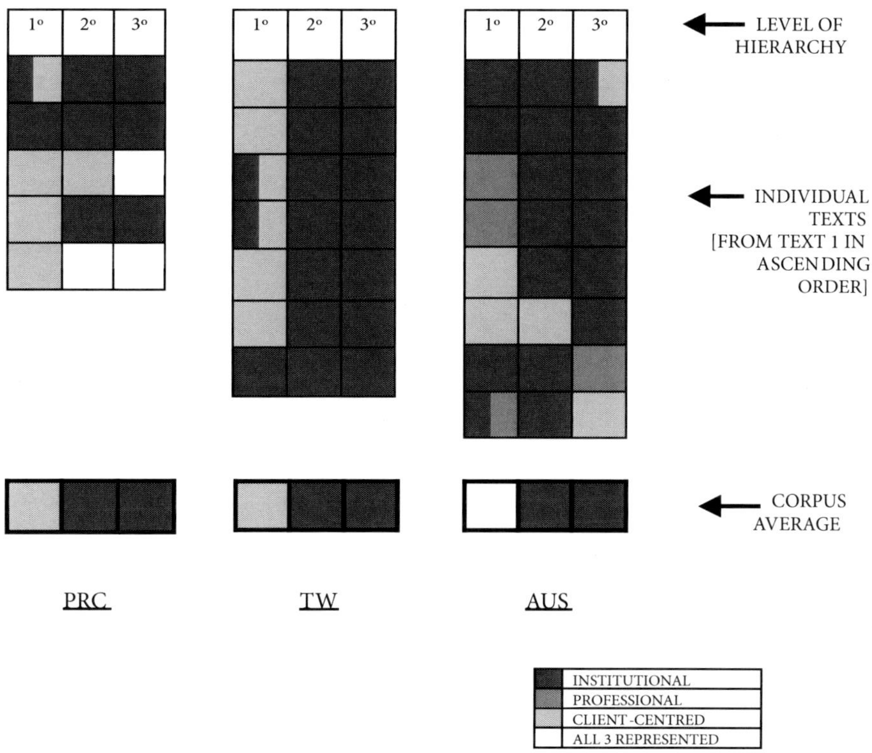

Figure 5.6 Comparison of discursive hierarchies across PRC, TW and AUS psychoeducational texts

The uniform resonance of the institutional voice across the psychoeducational corpora in terms of discursive content is replicated in their discursive hierarchies. Institutional discourse on average dominates the penultimate levels (secondary and tertiary) of the discursive hierarchy in all three corpora. Figure 5.6 shows that the institutional voice, in fact, resonates in at least one of the upper levels of the discursive hierarchy in all texts studied. The most common relations mediating this institutionality are solution and list, which are particularly widespread, followed by evaluation, motivation and antithesis. The pervasiveness of the solution relation can be explained by its capacity to "be a powerful and versatile persuasive tool" (Abelen, Redeker & Thompson 1993, p. 337), while lists represent an organisationally familiar and readily accessible format to the reader.

In only three individual texts across the three corpora, two from mainland China and one from Australia, does institutional discourse fail to dominate the upper levels of the text discursive hierarchy (see Figure 5.6). The upper hierarchies of these texts for the most part resonate the client-centred voice. The two

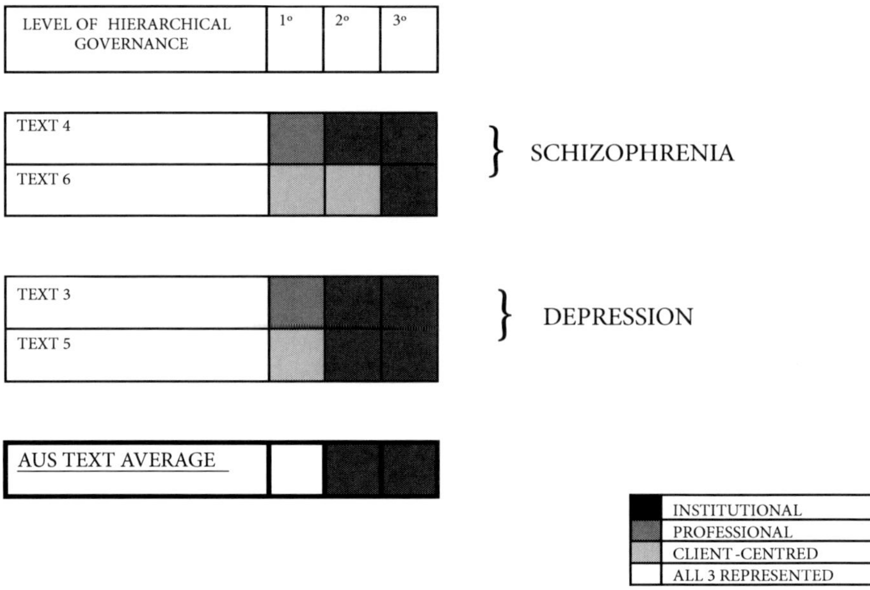

Figure 5.7 Variation in discursive hierarchy of AUS schizophrenia and depression texts

mainland Chinese texts are primarily narratives, hence their client-centred presentations. The Australian text, used for analytic demonstration in Chapter 4 of this volume, appears to acknowledge a perceived consumer preference for more client-centred representations of mental illness and mental health care.

While institutional discourse, on average, uniformly dominates the penultimate levels of the discursive hierarchies of all psychoeducational corpora, Figure 5.6 shows that the primary level of the discursive hierarchy differs across corpora. The typical indigenous Chinese text resonates the client-centred voice at this uppermost level. The most common relations mediating this client-centredness are elaboration and background. Similar to the findings obtained for discursive content in this study, empowerment does not feature in the discursive hierarchy of the indigenous Chinese psychoeducational texts. Unlike the indigenous Chinese texts, the primary level of the Australian texts resonates all three discursive voices. This variation at the uppermost level of the discursive hierarchy is not related to text topic, with individual schizophrenia and depression texts each resonating professional and client-centred voices at their primary levels (see Figure 5.7). Thus, mirroring the findings obtained for discursive content, the broader presentation of the Australian psychoeducational literature reflects the continuing debate in the West over preferred explanatory models of mental illness: biomedical versus client-centred (see Chapter 3, this volume). The most

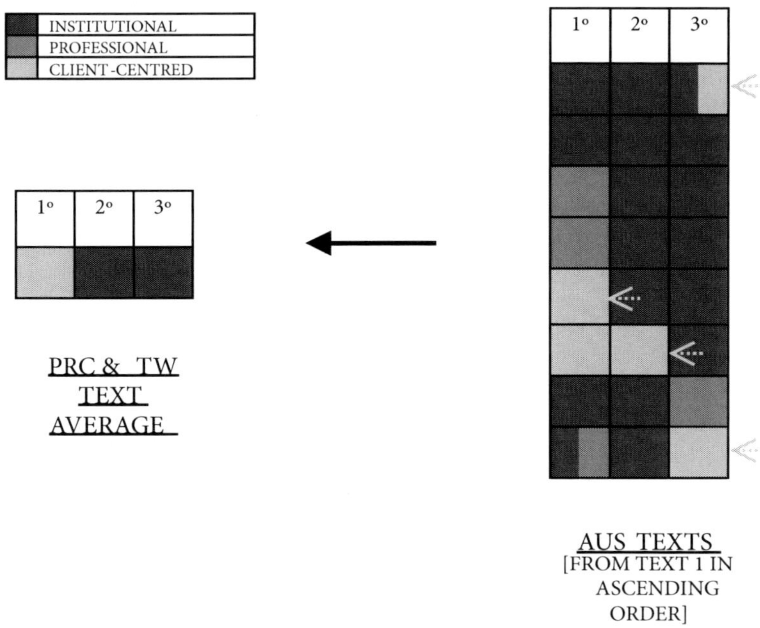

Figure 5.8 Discursive 'movement' in AUS psychoeducational texts

common relations mediating these presentations are conclusion (biomedical), where a finding can be logically inferred from preceding claims; and elaboration (client-centred), where the text provides additional details about subject matter.

Generally speaking, the discursive hierarchies of the psychoeducational literature under study, the more overt of the two discursive features analysed in this study, reflect the organisational context of text production and the preferred presentation of the texts. Indigenous Chinese texts are highly institutional in presentation to the reader and do not accentuate active empowerment. This adds weight to the earlier finding that normative communication of this type concurs with Confucian notions of direction by authority, unquestioning acceptance of fact and compliant response. This is what the mental health body perceives is appropriate to the circumstance and expected by the reader. The belief would be that providing otherwise might only confuse the reader. The Australian texts, on the other hand, while broadly institutional, possess a variety of overarching presentations. This diversity adds weight to the earlier claim that dominant society debate over preferred conceptions of mental illness and approaches to mental health care hegemonicly resonates in psychoeducational literature intended for Chinese-speaking migrants.

Figure 5.8 explains the aforementioned differences in the discursive hierarchies of indigenous Chinese and Australian psychoeducational corpora and the differences across individual texts comprising the Australian corpus in terms of discursive 'movement'. A growing acknowledgment of the client-centred voice, arising from promotion in the West of alternative conceptions of health in general and mental illness specifically, sees client-centredness steadily advance into the upper levels of discursive governance in the Australian texts, displacing the more traditional institutional and professional voices. Fulfilment of this trend ultimately would see the discursive hierarchies of indigenous Chinese and Australian psychoeducational corpora coincide. While ostensibly this could improve the communicative efficacy of the Australian psychoeducational message for Chinese-speaking migrants, differences in the nature of client-centredness across indigenous Chinese and Australian corpora also need to be considered. Greater resonance of consumer empowerment in psychoeducational literature targeting migrant Chinese in the end may lower communicative efficacy, given their cultural expectation for direction and instruction in these circumstances.

Communicating mental illness

The discussion undertaken in this chapter has explored similarities and differences in the discursive form of the Chinese-language psychoeducational literature analysed in this study. Analysis of the two discursive features explicated in Chapter 4 of this volume, discursive content, denoting the proportional resonance of salient voices, and discursive hierarchy, denoting the broader presentation to the reader, finds equivalence between mainland Chinese and Taiwanese corpora, contrary to expectations stated in the introductory chapter of this volume that disparate political and historical experiences (communist and colonial) may be of consequence here. It is believed that their similarity to a significant extent stems from (1) the salient influence of Confucian beliefs, which emphasise the heeding of authority and compliance; (2) communicative norms for persuasion in Chinese culture, which frequently draw on life experience; (3) understating of the professional voice of medicine, due to the potential intersection between the biomedical conception of mental illness and Chinese cultural stigma; and (4) shared organisational contexts of production.

The chapter has found that while an institutional core remains common to all corpora, reflecting the texts' organisational context of production, the discursive form of the Australian Chinese-language psychoeducational corpus differs in many ways from its indigenous Chinese counterparts. A hegemony of competing dominant culture conceptions of mental illness, one grounded in biomedicine and the other in notions of consumer empowerment, accounts for this finding. A potential intersection of Chinese stigmatic beliefs based on heredity with biomedical conceptions of mental illness also may account for the greater resonance of the professional voice of medicine in the Australian corpus when compared to its indigenous Chinese counterparts. In the context of Anglo-dominant Australian society, there exists no basis for this unfavourable intersection between psychoeducational message and culture-bound stigma, so dissemination of the preferred (professional) explanatory model of mental illness is much less problematic. The chapter determines that, owing to the differential formulation of the psychoeducational message across indigenous Chinese and migrant settings, the communicative efficacy of the Australian Chinese-language psychoeducational message may be compromised by a potentially discordant intersection with Chinese communicative norms and cultural expectations and by an unintended legitimisation of stigmatic features salient to Chinese cultural explanatory models.

Finally, the chapter has ascertained that disease topic can affect the discursive content of psychoeducational literature. Texts addressing schizophrenia and psychosis are more biomedicalised across all corpora while those addressing clinical depression are less so. This may reflect the greater social and cultural disembodiment that the delusions and hallucinations characterising schizophrenia and psychosis represent (see Chapter 3, this volume). Conversely, texts addressing clinical depression are more client-centred across all corpora. This may reflect a disease presentation that is more in tune with normative social behaviour and experience.

Interpositionings between all levels of Fairclough's model of discourse analysis presented in Chapter 3 of this volume have now been examined, namely: text, discursive practice and social practice. In addition, the final question pertaining to discourse analysis of 'multivocal' text, as raised in Chapter 3, has been addressed, namely: What meanings do the different voices contribute to producing? The preferred conception of mental illness (professional) and its intersection with prevailing cultural norms and lay conceptions of mental illness have been analysed. In the final chapter of this volume, the new insights into community psychoeducation across the Chinese diaspora presented in the current chapter are reflected on, both in terms of how these findings address the key issues relating to public health communication and cross-cultural communication raised in the introductory chapter of this volume as well as how they contribute to the theoretical understandings of medical discourse described in Chapter 3. Qualifications to the explanations proffered in the current chapter are also set forth, along with future research suggested by this study's findings.

CHAPTER 6

Conclusion

Community psychoeducation aims to shape the minds of a community toward a professional conception of mental illness. This volume has noted that reshaping community understandings of mental illness constitutes a particularly important strategy for improving health service engagement of, timely treatment of and prognostic outcomes for people with a mental illness. The volume has also shown that the heterogeneity characterising the cultural explanatory model of mental illness in Chinese societies, encompassing the ancestral, mystical, spiritual and somatic understandings of imperial times that still retain currency today, along with the nature of the intense stigma toward mental illness in Chinese societies that emerges from a Confucian emphasis on order and harmony and patrilineal continuity, mean that reshaping Chinese community understandings toward a professional explanatory model informed by biomedicine can be particularly problematic. There is a need, therefore, as recommended for any public health endeavour in the introductory chapter of this volume, to position culture as a primary consideration in the formulation of psychoeducational messages targeting Chinese speakers.

The heterogeneity characterising the Chinese cultural explanatory model of mental illness contrasts with the homogeneity of the professional explanatory model embraced across the globe. This volume has confirmed that the hegemonic dominance of the biomedical conception of mental illness, where disturbances in neurobiochemistry form the aetiological basis to the psychotic hallucinations and delusions characterising schizophrenia and the melancholy and fatigue characterising clinical depression, extends to psychiatric practice across the Chinese diaspora. Despite this hegemony of the biomedical conception, the professional voice of medicine, nevertheless, has been found to variably resonate in Chinese-language psychoeducational literature produced in indigenous Chinese and Western (migrant) settings. This finding in many ways echoes that found in the author's earlier studies of Chinese print mass media text (Ramsay 1997, 2000, 2001a, 2001b) where a globally uniform news text superstructural schema cloaks distinct differences in finer discursive features across Chinese and Western settings. Both findings ultimately foreground the salience of culture to communicative undertakings of any type. Accordingly, regardless of the hegemony of the biomedical conception of mental illness across global psychiatric practice, community psychoeducational messages formulated in indigenous Chinese settings continue to mediate features characterising normative persuasive communication in Chinese culture and take into account culture-bound stigmatic beliefs.

The indigenous Chinese psychoeducational literature analysed in this study is distinctively lifeworld in discursive form and downplays empowerment. The former corresponds to a discursive norm characterising persuasive communication in Chinese culture. Such a norm has precedence in traditional Chinese rhetoric (Lu 2000). Interestingly, prioritising life experience also characterises client-centred counter-discourse as promoted by many in the West in opposition to traditional medical approaches to health care. De-emphasis of empowerment accords with the Chinese cultural expectation for direction by authority and compliant response to instruction, as valorised in Confucian teachings (Ng 2000). This, however, does not tally with Western notions of client-centredness, which champion consumer empowerment.

The empowerment that is lacking in the indigenous Chinese psychoeducational literature, in contrast, is more evident in the Australian counterpart. This feature, along with greater resonance of the professional voice of medicine, distinguishes the Australian literature from the indigenous Chinese literature analysed in this study. Thus, biomedicalising mental illness and giving greater consideration to an active consumer role in the practice of mental health care, both deemed constructive albeit competing discursive strategies for community psychoeducation in Anglo-dominant Australian society, hegemonicly resonate in psychoeducational literature intended for Chinese-speaking migrants residing in Australia.

The volume has claimed that these differences in the discursive form of the indigenous Chinese and Australian psychoeducational messages may affect reception of the message by the migrant Chinese audience. There are three main bases to this claim. Firstly, culturally based communicative norms pertaining to health body advisory information such as that under study would likely lead Chinese speakers to expect direction and instruction to which they comply. Such expectation accords with Confucian emphasis on respect for authority, in particular learned authority. While a discursive profile mediating direction and compliance is evident in the indigenous Chinese psychoeducational literature, this is often not the case for the Australian literature targeting Chinese speaking migrants, where Anglo-dominant societal notions of empowerment appear to hegemonicly resonate in many instances. This may prove overly demanding on a Chinese speaking audience expecting direction.

A second discursive difference that may compromise the communicative efficacy of the Australian literature is its greater resonance of the professional voice of medicine. While biomedicalising mental illness remains a successful psychoeducational strategy in Anglo-dominant society, this volume has made clear that such a strategy may be counterproductive for a Chinese-speaking audience, given the biogenetic component to culture-bound stigma which sees mental illness as running in family lines. Here, as evidenced in Gallois and Callan's (1997) study of HIV/AIDS community education programs in Africa, cited in the introductory chapter of this volume, discursive strategies deemed effective for Western audiences do not necessarily prove effective for other cultural groups.

Thirdly, greater resonance of the voice of the lifeworld in the indigenous Chinese texts, deemed a successful strategy for persuasive communication in Chinese cultural contexts, may see the psychoeducational message more effectively conveyed in the mainland Chinese and Taiwanese psychoeducational literature when compared to their Australian counterpart. The volume has noted that greater reference to life experience in public health communication is likely to prove beneficial in all cultural settings and, indeed, there appears to be acknowledgment of this in individual Australian texts studied. Greater resonance of the voice of the lifeworld is viewed by many in the West as a client-centred initiative that counters the professional and institutional discursive biases traditionally deemed to characterise medical communication. The findings of this study where individual psychoeducational texts feature lifeworld discursive forms in tandem with institutional forms, however, appear to support research findings that caution that lifeworld forms can be re-articulated in institutional communication in order to achieve institutionally derived goals that were previously achieved by overtly authoritative use of language. The strategic 'conversationalisation' of texts produced by organisations and an increasing use of narrative in advertising in the West illustrate a trend where utilisation of the lifeworld voice in the end merely serves as "further camouflage for introducing new forms of public control" (Sarangi & Slembrouck 1996, p. 9). Care, therefore, needs to be taken in unequivocally interpreting the client-centredness explicated in the psychoeducational texts under study as manifesting the goals of the latter-day consumer empowerment movement in the West, given that "the lifeworld (of conversations, informality and day to day shopping) and the system world (of institutions, formality and red tape) … now share common discursive practices" (Sarangi & Roberts 1999, p. 33).

An important caveat to this volume arises from evaluating the potential communicative efficacy of the Chinese-language psychoeducational texts under study under the assumption that the indigenous Chinese texts effectively communicate the intended message. Premising this volume is a recommendation for more effective community psychoeducation targeting Chinese speaking migrants residing in multicultural countries such as Australia and the United States. The introductory chapter of the volume has noted that such a recommendation stems from numerous studies that have documented strikingly lower use of mental health services and higher involuntary hospital admissions for Chinese speaking migrants residing in Western countries, in particular when compared to the locally-born population but also when compared to co-resident migrant groups (Fan & Karnilowicz 2000; Klimidis, et al. 1999a, 1999b; Kung 2001; Loo, Tong & True 1989; Minas, et al. 1996; Sue & Morishima 1982; Tabora & Flaskerud 1997). Improved community psychoeducation, along with a range of health service access and equity measures, are viewed as necessary responses in addressing these usage and admission issues (Chiu 1987).

The discursive differences that distinguish the psychoeducational texts targeting Chinese speaking migrants from those produced in indigenous Chinese settings indicate that the Australian texts are less likely to successfully convey the intended message when compared to their indigenous Chinese counterparts. This is because discursive features characterising the indigenous Chinese psychoeducational literature are readily accounted for by cultural phenomena salient to the Chinese experience. A close correspondence between mainland Chinese and Taiwanese psychoeducational literature, despite the disparate political and social histories of mainland China and Taiwan, further points to the salient impact of culture. The discursive features characterising the Australian Chinese-language literature, in contrast, appear to reflect phenomena salient to Anglo-dominant society. Thus, being more culturally responsive, it would be expected that the indigenous Chinese psychoeducational literature would be more effective in communicating the intended message. Moreover, greater consideration of cultural phenomena by public health bodies engaged in community psychoeducation targeting Chinese speaking migrants would be expected to improve communication of the intended psychoeducational message and so contribute to addressing the service usage and hospital admission concerns raised earlier.

Although the volume has uncovered cultural specificity in the discursive form of the psychoeducation literature, which sees analogous forms present in disparate indigenous settings, there nevertheless remains no direct evidence that the culturally preferred discursive form is more conducive to effective communication. Chapter 2 of this volume noted that in mainland China eighty percent of people with a serious mental illness are believed to receive no treatment at all for their disorder, a much higher proportion than, for example, in Australia (Pearson 1996; Ran, et al. 2005). The chapter also noted that a large percentage of people with a mental illness in mainland China and Taiwan primarily consult folk healers for treatment. The grim mental health service treatment statistics appear to suggest that community psychoeducation in mainland China and Taiwan is *less* effective than that provided for Chinese speaking migrants residing in Australia, contrary to claims presented in this study that point to the cultural appropriateness of the indigenous Chinese psychoeducational literature. However, economic considerations present a major obstacle to contact with health services in mainland China and Taiwan where all services, including mental health care, are provided on a user-pay basis, unlike Australia where a national health scheme provides universal coverage for all residents and, in particular, where government in-patient and community mental health services are provided free of charge (Ran, et al. 2005). It remains rather problematic, therefore, to evaluate the success of community psychoeducation in mainland China and Taiwan due to these overriding access and equity concerns.

Although uncertainty exists as to the actual communicative efficacy of the mainland Chinese and Taiwanese psychoeducational literature, this volume nevertheless has explicated clear discursive differences between the indigenous Chinese literature and their Australian counterpart, which point to a greater cultural responsiveness of the former. Those seeking to improve the communicative efficacy of the Australian literature targeting Chinese speaking migrants, whose effectiveness has been brought into question by a number of studies, are encouraged, therefore, to consider conclusions made in this study stemming from the explicated differences in discursive form in psychoeducational literature produced in indigenous Chinese and Western (migrant) settings. By definition, the role of discourse analysis is not to solve the communicative dilemma; discourse analysis first and foremost constitutes "a tool which is used … to identify limitations of as well as desirable alternatives to current discursive practices" (Willig 1999, p. 149). The limitations of current discursive practice in the literature in question have been clearly identified in this volume. It remains the province of other disciplinary investigators, here communication researchers, to empirically evaluate the communicative consequences of the discourse analytic findings made in this study and propose remedies based thereon.

The analysis undertaken in this volume also further contributes to understanding medical discourse and methodological means for examining its make-up. The RST framework has been confirmed as a useful discourse analytic tool for analysing public health literature, analysing texts written in non-European language, and ascertaining in what manner and to what extent discursive voices deemed salient to medical communication resonate in public health literature. The framework's ability to attend to hierarchy as well as scale has allowed this study to deliver a more comprehensive analysis than alternative discourse analytic approaches based on selective commentary and confined to subject-matter-based determinations neglecting hierarchy. Fairclough's discourse analytic model, which posits an inter-positioning of text, discursive practice and social practice, too, has been shown to provide a useful heuristic for "research on communication and society" of this type (Jørgensen & Phillips 2002, p. 69).

The hybrid nature of medical discourse has been substantiated in this volume, along with the more nuanced discursive distinction between the professional voice, mediating expert knowledge and specialised practice, and the institutional voice, mediating control and the setting of rules and boundaries, as espoused by Sarangi and Roberts amongst others. This is similarly the case for the client-centred voice, characterised by Mishler's voice of the lifeworld and latter-day notions of consumer empowerment. Together, these discursive voices provide a conceptual framework of high explanatory value for the phenomena of interest to this study, thus confirming the soundness of their "delimitation" for analysis of medical discourse (Jørgensen & Phillips 2002, p. 144). The volume explicated in some psychoeducational texts, as mentioned earlier, a hybrid articulation between lifeworld and institutional voices, which likely sees the former appropriated to achieve organisation goals. Jørgensen and Phillips (2002, p. 73) note that articulations of discourses "in new and complex ways – in new 'interdiscursive mixes' – are both a sign of, and a driving force in, discursive and thereby socio-cultural change." Discursive articulations explicated in this volume, however, in the end appear to only serve to sustain "the stability of the dominant order of discourse and thereby the dominant social order" (Jørgensen & Phillips 2002, p. 73). That is, while use of the lifeworld voice can bring the intended message closer to the consumer's frame of day-to-day experience, a concomitant institutional dominance of the discursive hierarchy in many texts studied here suggest that the use of the lifeworld voice merely serves to screen the authoritative voice of the institution and, as such, facilitate maintenance of the authoritative position of the public health body.

It is worth reminding the reader that the volume ultimately makes no specific claims as to the intentionality of the writer/s of the texts in producing texts with a particular discursive makeup. The vocal arrangements explicated in the texts under study reflect discursive positionings and, as such, embody how certain ways of representing the world – professional, institutional, client-centred – are realised in and constituted by texts. A discursive feature of a text may reflect a calculated strategy by the text writer/s or may simply reflect the natural expression of a certain way of representing aspects of the world. Use of the lifeworld voice as a communicative norm for persuasion in an indigenous Chinese text may register lower on the intentionality scale while its use to camouflage institutional goals in an Australian text may register higher on such a scale. Such judgements, however, are open to contention and remain beyond the immediate scope of this study. What is demonstrated in this volume, however, is that these discursive features exist, they have explanation and they have potential consequences in relation to the communicative efficacy of the texts concerned.

In addition to its analytic findings and their implications for communication research, an important contribution of this volume has been its assembling in one source a widely-dispersed body of research examining traditional and contemporary conceptions of mental illness in Chinese societies. Chapter 2 has revealed a complexity of lay understandings of mental illness and of pathways to mental health care in Chinese societies. The chapter has also revealed the focal position of family in Chinese societies, which sees them play a key role in responding to mental illness when it appears in a family member and in choosing from amongst a range of pathways to care available in Chinese societies. This situation serves to emphasise the importance of effective community psychoeducation in Chinese societies so that informed family members respond appropriately when mental illness arises within the family (Fan & Karnilowicz 2000; Pearson & Phillips 1994; Ran, et al. 2003, 2005; Zhang, et al. 1993). Chapter 2 confirmed a dominance of the biomedical conception of mental illness amongst mainland Chinese and Taiwanese health professionals. Community psychoeducation in mainland China and Taiwan, therefore, would seek to reshape lay thinking toward mental illness away from a plurality of understandings toward a homogenous biomedical conception. While shaping community thinking in such a direction would assist public health bodies in their management of mental health care, the volume has also noted congruence between the biomedical conception and the mainland Chinese government's eugenic vision for a healthy and 'high-quality' population, which is disseminated in particular through the one-child campaign for population control. This eugenic vision propagates the undesirability of mental illness and links it directly to heredity. Greater lay acceptance of the biomedical explanatory model arising from successful community psychoeducation in mainland China, while seen by health professionals to provide for better health care outcomes for people with a mental illness, at the same time risks affirming a government sponsored eugenic vision that has obvious negative consequences for people with a mental illness. A similar danger exists across all Chinese societies given the biogenetic component to cultural stigma. Thus, this volume cautions that an explanatory model of mental illness which aims to improve the lives of, provide better health care outcomes for and reduce community stigma toward people with a mental illness, on the contrary, may see people with a mental illness further stigmatised as lacking in biological 'quality' and further victimised through legislated or social exclusion from the reproductive pool. Great care must be taken, therefore, when applying public health strategies deemed of universal benefit to global populations to specific social and cultural contexts.

A wider-reaching finding of this volume, whose implications extend beyond the specific linguistic and cultural borders of the psychoeducational literature under study, is the difference in discursive form of texts addressing schizophrenia and psychosis when compared to those addressing mental illness generically or other specific disorders such as clinical depression. The greater resonance of the professional voice of medicine in texts addressing schizophrenia and psychosis from *all* corpora likely reflects a disease symptomatology that particularly challenges societal norms of behaviour. Such a confronting disorder is universally rationalised, it seems, by greater foregrounding of a biomedical conception. A perceived need for such a strategy in relation to community psychoeducation about schizophrenia and psychosis, drawing heavily on bioscience while retreating from the lifeworld, highlights that the depth of stigma toward the disease is apparent in the communicative behaviour of those seeking to overcome this phenomenon. The very perception by public health educators of a need to represent this disorder so differently from mental illness generically or other specific disorders such as clinical depression reinforces the extent to which schizophrenia and psychosis are conceived of as highly marginalised, socially disruptive and, for many, dangerous disease experiences. This is further accentuated by the distinctive discursive form of psychoeducational texts addressing clinical depression in this study, a disorder that falls more within the frame of normative human experience, where texts appear more 'at ease' in voicing the lifeworld.

Specifically, returning to the Chinese experience, such findings echo claims by Pearson (1995c) that Chinese people demonstrate great tolerance for depressive symptomatology but little for psychosis. This arises, as noted in Chapter 2 of this volume, from the strong association of psychosis in Chinese culture with disorder of the mind, which is not the case for depression. Given that Chiu (1987, p. 10) states that Chinese people "cannot easily accept a primary disorder of thought" as it portends loss of control of revered human and social attributes such as propriety, moral judgment, harmony and order, Chinese community psychoeducation about schizophrenia will always present a great challenge to public health bodies.

In approaching the close of this volume, it is important to keep in mind that while many positions argued in this and related volumes seemingly are highly critical of the hegemony of the biomedical explanatory model of health and illness amongst health professionals as well as across many societies across the globe, the study does not wish to diminish the many benefits that such a conception can bring to the practice of mental health care. It is not biomedical science that is contested by research of this type, but its often hegemonic dominance to the exclusion of alternative understandings. The findings of this volume caution mental health bodies of the attendant dangers of overstatement of the biomedical explanatory model when undertaking community psychoeducation targeting Chinese speakers. It would be unfortunate if such cautioning, however, led to silencing of the professional voice of medicine in psychoeducational and other public health endeavours. As Kim (2003, p. 443) states:

> The criticisms raised by … critics of scientific epistemology do not deny the value of the rational, inferential knowledge. Rather, they are directed to the error of Western philosophy in regarding concepts that do not adhere to its mode as invalid. They refer to the arrogance or overconfidence in believing that scientific knowledge is the only way to discover truth, when, in reality, the very process of doing science requires an immediate, aesthetic experience of the phenomenon under investigation.

This volume, therefore, calls for a balanced position that acknowledges the value of the biomedical conception of health and illness but does not see it dominate to the detriment of the unwell. For example, a great deal can be lost by ascribing to the unwell a wholly biomedically derived "attribution of 'deviance'" whereby "they stop being seen in terms of individual cases, and come to represent very menacing forms of *collective* adversity which threaten the equilibrium of the whole community" [original emphasis] (Rogers 1991, p. 37). Equally, the volume calls for a balanced position whereby health consumers make determinations as to how to conceptualise illness, in ways which are in harmony with understandings gained through life experience yet which, at the same time, do not deny access to contemporary treatment options, many biomedical, that may significantly improve their quality of life. In this balanced discursive position, Rogers (1991, p. 39) states,

> the medical establishment is able to recognize the ideological traps of reification, medicalization and the dogmatic assumption that 'we know best', and yet is not so paralysed by these challenges to its basic tenets that it becomes unable to deal effectively with biological catastrophes.

There is little to be gained by "romanticising patients and demonising medicine by the "patient empowerment" discourse" if this ultimately leads to negative outcomes for people with a mental illness and their carers by merely dissuading them from seeking to engage with potentially effective medical therapeutic options (Dixon-Woods 2001, p. 1427).

The introductory chapter of this volume highlighted that in order to effectively communicate a public health message it is imperative to locate culture as a key consideration in the communicative undertaking. Findings of this volume suggest that cultural considerations are evident in the mainland Chinese and Taiwanese psychoeducational literature under study but less so in the Australian Chinese-language counterpart. The indigenous Chinese texts, it appears, heed the advice of Kuo and Kavanagh (1994, p. 554) that

> When it is necessary for aspects of Western biomedicine or health care to intrude upon traditional ideas, that intervention will be least resisted when the integrity of familiar, culturally oriented beliefs and behaviors is maintained … For example, explanations can be given in ways that fit clients' expectations.

The Australian texts do not appear to meet such expectations. While the volume has noted reservations as to the communicative efficacy of the mainland Chinese and Taiwanese psychoeducational literature, their distinct differences in discursive form when compared to the Australian Chinese-language counterpart suggests a greater degree of cultural resonance in the mainland Chinese and Taiwanese literature. Commonality in message form and reader expectation would likely heighten the efficacy of message communication in the mainland Chinese and Taiwanese psychoeducational literature (Bhui & Rüdell 2002; Kua, Chew & Ko 1993; Witte & Morrison 1995). As such, this literature may be a suitable prototype for Western counterparts targeting migrant communities, such as the Australian psychoeducational literature under study.

The importance of such a finding to the quest to effectively deliver appropriate mental health care and services to Chinese speakers across the globe cannot be understated. As Wodak (1996, p. 35) states, "the risk for the medical institution is that ineffectual communication will lead to harmful consequences". These consequences for people with a mental illness and their families are ever agonising and distressing, particularly in the case of Chinese speakers, and they have been left unaddressed for far too long.

Bibliography

Abelen, E., Redeker, G. & Thompson, S. A. 1993. The rhetorical structure of US-American and Dutch fund-raising letters. *Text*, 13 (3), 323–350.

Agar, M. 1985. Institutional discourse. *Text*, 5 (3), 147–168.

Ainsworth-Vaughn, N. 2003. The discourse of medical encounters. In D. Schiffrin, D. Tannen & H. E. Hamilton (eds.) *The handbook of discourse analysis* (pp. 453–469). Oxford: Blackwell.

Arthur, V. A. M. 1995. Written patient information: A review of the literature. *Journal of Advanced Nursing*, 21 (6), 1081–1086.

Azar, M. 1999. Argumentative text as rhetorical structure: An application of rhetorical structure theory. *Argumentation*, 13 (1), 97–114.

Bahl, V. 1999. Mental illness: A national perspective. In D. Bhugra & V. Bahl (eds.) *Ethnicity: An agenda for mental health* (pp. 7–22). Gaskell: The Royal College of Psychiatrists.

Barton, E. 2000. Sanctioned and non-sanctioned narratives in institutional discourse. *Narrative Inquiry*, 10 (20), 341–375.

Bentelspacher, C. E., Chitran, S. & Rahman, M. B. A. 1994. Coping and adaptation patterns among Chinese, Indian, and Malay families caring for a mentally ill relative. *Families in Society*, 75 (5), 287–294.

Bhugra, D., Lippett, R. & Cole, E. 1999. Pathways into care: An explanation of the factors that may affect minority ethnic groups. In D. Bhugra & V. Bahl (eds.) *Ethnicity: An agenda for mental health* (pp. 29–39). Gaskell: The Royal College of Psychiatrists.

Bhui, K. & Bhugra, D. 2002. Explanatory models for mental distress: Implications for clinical practice and research. *The British Journal of Psychiatry*, 181, 6–7.

Bhui, K. & Rüdell, K. 2002. Transcultural mental health promotion. *Journal of Mental Health Promotion*, 1 (1), 8–15.

Boey, K. W. 1997. Help-seeking pattern of psychiatric outpatients in urban China. *The International Journal of Psychiatric Nursing Research*, 4 (1), 433–443.

Brassington, C. 1995. *The portrayal of disability in contemporary Chinese literature and its relationship to perceptions of and attitudes towards people with disabilities in contemporary Chinese society: An investigative study*. Unpublished doctoral dissertation. University of Queensland.

Callan, A. & Littlewood, R. 1998. Patient satisfaction: Ethnic origin or explanatory model? *International Journal of Social Psychiatry*, 44 (1), 1–11.

Candlin, C. N. 2001. Medical discourse as professional and institutional action: Challenges to teaching and researching languages for special purposes. In M. Bax & C. J. Zwart (eds.) *Reflections on language and language learning: In honour of Arthur Van Essen* (pp. 185–207). Amsterdam: John Benjamins.

Cheung, F. M. 1995. Facts and myths about somatization among the Chinese. In T. Lin, W. Tseng & E. Yeh (eds.) *Chinese society and mental health* (pp. 156–166). Hong Kong: Oxford University Press.

Chiu, L. P. W. 1987. Educating Chinese schizophrenic patients about their illness. *Hong Kong Journal of Mental Health*, 16, 6–13.

Chiu, M. L. 1981. Insanity in imperial China: A legal case study. In A. Kleinman & T. Lin (eds.) *Normal and abnormal behaviour in Chinese culture* (pp. 75–94). Dordrecht; Boston: D. Reidel.

Chiu, M. L. 1986. *Mind, body, and illness in a Chinese medical tradition*. Unpublished doctoral dissertation. Ann Arbor, MI: University Microfilms International.

Committee on Communication for Behavior Change in the 21st Century: Improving the Health of Diverse Populations. 2002. *Speaking of health: Assessing health communication strategies for diverse populations*. Washington, DC: The National Academies Press.

Commonwealth Department of Health and Aged Care. 1999. *Mental health promotion and prevention: National action plan under the second national mental health plan: 1998–2003*. Canberra: Promotion and Prevention Section, Mental Health Branch, Commonwealth Department of Health and Aged Care.

Cora-Brambel, D. & Williams, L. 2000. Explaining illness to Latinos: Cultural foundations and messages. In B. B. Whaley (ed.) *Explaining illness: Research, theory, and strategies* (pp. 257–280). Mahwah: Lawrence Erlbaum Associates.

Cottrell, R. R., Girvan, J. T. & McKenzie, J. F. 2002. *Principles and foundations of health promotion and education*. San Francisco: Benjamin Cummings.

Coulter, A. 1998. Evidence based patient information. *BMJ*, 317, 225–226.

Coulter, A., Entwistle, V. & Gilbert, D. 1998. *Informing patients: An assessment of the quality of patient information materials*. London: King's Fund.

Coupland, J., Robinson, J. D. & Coupland, N. 1994. Frame negotiation in doctor-elderly patient consultations. *Discourse and Society*, 5 (1), 89–124.

Dikötter, F. 1998. *Imperfect conceptions: Medical knowledge, birth defects and eugenics in China*. London: Hurst & Co.

Dixon, L., Adams, C. & Lucksted, A. 2000. Update on family psychoeducation for schizophrenia. *Schizophrenia Bulletin*, 26 (1), 5–20.

Dixon-Woods, M. 2001. Writing wrongs? An analysis of published discourses about the use of patient information leaflets. *Social Science and Medicine*, 52, 1417–1432.

Edelstein, A. S., Ito, Y. & Kepplinger, H. M. 1989. *Communication and culture: A comparative approach*. New York: Longman.

Fairclough, N. 2003. *Analysing discourse: Textual analysis for social research*. London; New York: Routledge.

Fan, C. & Karnilowicz, W. 2000. Attitudes towards mental illness and knowledge of mental health services among the Australian and Chinese community. *Australian Journal of Primary Health*, 6 (2), 38–48.

Fisher, S. & Todd, A. D. 1986a. Introduction: Communication in institutional contexts: Social interaction and social structure. In S. Fisher & A. D. Todd (eds.) *Discourse and institutional authority: Medicine, education, and law* (pp. ix–xviii). Norwood, NJ: Ablex.

Fisher, S. & Todd, A. D. 1986b. Friendly persuasion: Negotiating decisions to use oral contraceptives. In S. Fisher & A. D. Todd (eds.) *Discourse and institutional authority: Medicine, education, and law* (pp. 3–25). Norwood, NJ: Ablex.

Fleischman, S. 2003. Language and medicine. In D. Schiffrin, D. Tannen & H. E. Hamilton (eds.) *The handbook of discourse analysis* (pp. 470–502). Oxford: Blackwell.

Fox, B. A. 1987. *Discourse structure and anaphora: Written and conversational English*. Cambridge: Cambridge University Press.

Fraser, J. 1999. The discourse of official texts and how it can impede public service translators. *Journal of Multilingual and Multicultural Development*, 20 (3), 194– 208.

Fries, P. H. 1994. On theme, rheme and discourse goals. In M. Coulthard (ed.) *Advances in written text analysis* (pp. 229–249). London: Routledge.

Furnham, A. & Malik, R. 1994. Cross-cultural beliefs about "depression". *The International Journal of Social Psychiatry*, 40 (2), 106–123.

Gallois, C. & Callan, V. J. 1997. *Communication and culture: A guide for practice*. Chichester: John Wilely & Sons.

Garcés, C. V. 2002. Translation and stereotypes as cultural facts: A case study, AIDS and the Latino community in the USA. *Babel*, 48 (4), 289–304.

Garcés, C. V. 2005. Doctor-patient consultations in dyadic and triadic exchanges. *Interpreting*, 7(2), 193–210.

Garro, L. C. & Mattingly, C. 2000a. Narrative as construct and construction. In C. Mattingly & L. C. Garro (eds.) *Narrative and the cultural construction of illness and healing* (pp. 1–49). Berkeley, CA: University of California Press.

Garro, L. C. & Mattingly, C. 2000b. Narrative turns. In C. Mattingly & L. C. Garro (eds.) *Narrative and the cultural construction of illness and healing* (pp. 259–270). Berkeley, CA: University of California Press.

Gee, J. P. 1999. *An introduction to discourse analysis: Theory and method*. New York: Routledge.

Geist-Martin, P., Ray, E. B. & Sharf, B. F. 2003. *Communicating health: Personal, cultural, and political complexities*. Belmont, CA: Thomson/Wadsworth.

Gwyn, R. 2002. *Communicating health and illness*. London: Sage Publications.

Harper. D. J. 1995. Discourse analysis and 'mental health'. *Journal of Mental Health*, 4, 347–357.

Harper. D. J. 1996. Deconstructing 'Paranoia': Towards a discursive understanding of apparently unwarranted suspicion. *Theory and Psychology*, 6 (3), 423–448.

Harper, D. 1999. Tablet talk and depot discourse: Discourse analysis and psychiatric medication. In C. Willig (ed.) *Applied discourse analysis: Social and psychological interventions* (pp. 125–144). Buckingham: Open University Press.

Harris, S. 2003. Politeness and power: Making and responding to 'requests' in institutional settings. *Text*, 23 (1), 27–52.

He, A. W. 1998. *Reconstructing institutions: Language use in academic counselling encounters*. Greenwich, CT: Ablex.

Hsueh-Shih, C. Development of mental health systems and care in China: From the 1940s through the 1980s. In T. Lin, W. Tseng & E. Yeh (eds.) *Chinese society and mental health* (pp. 315–325). Hong Kong: Oxford University Press.

Iedema, R. 1997. The language of administration: Organizing human activity in formal institutions. In F. Christie & J. R. Martin (eds.) *Genre and institutions: Social processes in the workplace and school* (pp. 73–118). London: Cassell.

Iedema, R. 2003. *Discourses of post-bureaucratic organization*. Amsterdam; Philadelphia: John Benjamins.

Jacobs, G. 1995. Organization in institutional discourse: Putting press releases on a proper footing. In B. Wårvik, S. Tanskanen & R. Hiltunen (eds.) *Organization in discourse: Proceedings from the Turku Conference (Anglicana Turkuensia 14)* (pp. 301–307). 10–14 August, 1994, Turku, Finland.

Jandt, F. E. 2004. *An introduction to intercultural communication: Identities in a global community*. Thousand Oaks: Sage Publications.

Jaworski, A. & Coupland, N. 1999. Introduction: Perspectives on discourse analysis. In A. Jaworski & N. Coupland (eds.) *The discourse reader* (pp. 1–44). London; New York: Routledge.

Johnson, F. L. 2003. Cultural dimensions of discourse. In L. A. Samovar & R. E. Porter (eds.) *Intercultural communication: A reader* (pp. 184–197). Belmont, CA: Wadsworth/Thomson Learning.

Jørgensen, M. & Phillips, L. 2002. *Discourse analysis: As theory and method*. London: Sage Publications.

Kim, Y. Y. 2003. Intercultural personhood: An integration of Eastern and Western perspectives. In L. A. Samovar & R. E. Porter (eds.) *Intercultural communication: A reader* (pp. 436–448). Belmont, CA: Wadsworth/Thomson Learning.

King, A. Y. C. & Bond, M. H. 1985. The Confucian paradigm of man: A sociological view. In W. Tseng & D. Y. H. Wu (eds.) *Chinese culture and mental health* (pp. 29–46). London: Academic Press.

Kirkpatrick, A. 1993. Information sequencing in Modern Standard Chinese. *Australian Review of Applied Linguistics*, 16 (2), 27–60.

Kleinman, A. 1980. *Patients and healers in the context of culture: An exploration of the borderland between anthropology, medicine, and psychiatry*. Berkeley, CA: University of California Press.

Kleinman, A. 1986. *Social origins of distress and disease: Depression, neurasthenia, and pain in modern China*. New Haven; London: Yale University Press.

Kleinman, A. & Kleinman, J. 1995. Remembering the Cultural Revolution: Alienating pains and the pain of alienation/transformation. In T. Lin, W. Tseng & E. Yeh (eds.) *Chinese society and mental health* (pp. 141–155). Hong Kong: Oxford University Press.

Kleinman, A. & Mechanic, D. 1981. Mental illness and psychosocial aspects of medical problems in China. In A. Kleinman & T. Lin (eds.) *Normal and abnormal behaviour in Chinese culture* (pp. 331–356). Dordrecht; Boston: D. Reidel.

Klimidis, S., Lewis, J., Miletic, T., McKenzie, S., Stolk, Y. & Minas, H. 1999a. *Mental health service use by ethnic communities in Victoria: Part I*. Melbourne: Victorian Transcultural Psychiatry Unit and Centre for Cultural Studies in Health.

Klimidis, S., Lewis, J., Miletic, T., McKenzie, S., Stolk, Y. & Minas, H. 1999b. *Mental health service use by ethnic communities in Victoria: Part II: Statistical tables*. Melbourne: Victorian Transcultural Psychiatry Unit and Centre for Cultural Studies in Health.

Kong, K. C. C. 1998. Are simple business request letters really simple? A comparison of Chinese and English business request letters. *Text*, 18 (1), 103–141.

Kua, E. H., Chew, P. H. & Ko, S. M. 1993. Spirit possession and healing among Chinese psychiatric patients. *Acta Psychiatrica Scandinavica*, 88, 447–450.

Kung, W. W. 2001. Consideration of cultural factors in working with Chinese American families with a mentally ill patient. *The Journal of Contemporary Human Services*, 82 (1), 97–107.

Kuo, C. L. & Kavanagh, K. H. 1994. Chinese perspectives on culture and mental health. *Issues in Mental Health Nursing*, 15, 551–567.

Leff, J. 1999. Epidemiological factors in research with ethnic minorities. In D. Bhugra & V. Bahl (eds.) *Ethnicity: An agenda for mental health* (pp. 40–47). Gaskell: The Royal College of Psychiatrists.

Lehtonen, M. 2000. *Cultural analysis of texts* (Translated by A. Ahonen and K. Clarke). London: Sage Publications.

Leung, J. P. 1998. Emotions and mental health in Chinese people. *Journal of Child and Family Studies*, 7 (2), 115–128.

Li, S. & Phillips, M. R. 1990. Witch doctors and mental illness in mainland China: A preliminary study. *The American Journal of Psychiatry*, 147 (2), 221–224.

Lin, K. 1981. Traditional Chinese medical beliefs and their relevance for mental illness and psychiatry. In A. Kleinman & T. Lin (eds.) *Normal and abnormal behaviour in Chinese culture* (pp. 95–114). Dordrecht; Boston: D. Reidel.

Lin, K., Kleinman, A. & Lin T. 1981. Overview of mental disorders in Chinese cultures: Review of epidemiological and clinical studies. In A. Kleinman & T. Lin (eds.) *Normal and abnormal behaviour in Chinese culture* (pp. 237–272). Dordrecht; Boston: D. Reidel.

Lin, T. 1982. Culture and psychiatry: A Chinese perspective. *Australian and New Zealand Journal of Psychiatry*, 16, 235–245.

Lin, T. 1985. Mental disorders and psychiatry in Chinese culture: Characteristic features and major issues. In W. Tseng & D. Y. H. Wu (eds.) *Chinese culture and mental health* (pp. 369–390). London: Academic Press.

Lin, T. & Lin, M. 1981. Love, denial and rejection: Responses of Chinese families to mental illness. In A. Kleinman & T. Lin (eds.) *Normal and abnormal behaviour in Chinese culture* (pp. 387–402). Dordrecht; Boston: D. Reidel.

Lin, T., Tseng, W. & Yeh, E. 1995. Chinese culture, orientation, and coping. In T. Lin, W. Tseng & E. Yeh (eds.) *Chinese society and mental health* (pp. 1–2). Hong Kong: Oxford University Press.

Long, H., Pirkis, J., Mihalopoulos, C., Narcarella, L., Summers, M. & Dunt, D. 1999. *Evaluating mental health service frameworks for non-English speaking background communities*. Melbourne: Australian Transcultural Mental Health Network.

Loo, C., Tong, B. & True, R. 1989. A bitter bean: Mental health status and attitudes in Chinatown. *Journal of Community Psychology*, 17, 283–295.

Lu, X. 1972. A madman's diary. In X. Lu *Selected stories of Lu Hsun* (pp. 7–18). Peking: Foreign Languages Press.

Lu, X. 2000. The influence of classical Chinese rhetoric on contemporary Chinese political communication and social relations. In D. R. Heisey (ed.) *Chinese perspectives in rhetoric and communication* (pp. 3–24). Stamford: Ablex.

Lupton, D. 1992. Discourse analysis: A new methodology for understanding the ideologies of health and illness. *Australian Journal of Public Health*, 16 (2), 145–149.

McCabe, R. & Priebe, S. 2004. Explanatory models of illness in schizophrenia: Comparison of four ethnic groups. *British Journal of Psychiatry*, 185, 25–30.

McCulloch, A. 1998. Public education in England. In R. Jenkins & T. B. Üstün (eds.) *Preventing mental illness: Mental health promotion in primary care* (pp. 269–276). Chichester: John Wiley & Sons.

MacDonald, M. N. 2002. Pedagogy, pathology and ideology: The production, transmission and reproduction of medical discourse. *Discourse and Society*, 13 (4), 447–467.

MacDonald, T. H. 1998. *Rethinking health promotion: A global approach*. London; New York: Routledge.

McDougall, B. & Louie, K. 1997. *The literature of China in the twentieth century*. London: Hurst & Co.

McGrath, J., Saha, S., Welham, J., El Saadi, O., MacCauley, C. & Chant, D. 2004. A systematic review of the incidence of schizophrenia: The distribution of rates and the influence of sex, urbanicity, migrant status and methodology. *BMC Medicine*, 2 (13), 1–22. doi:10.1186/1741-7015-2-13.

Mann, W. C. & Matthiessen. C. M. I. M. 1991. Functions of language in two frameworks. *Word*, 42, 231–249.

Mann, W. C., Matthiessen, C. M. I. M & Thompson, S. A. 1992. Rhetorical Structure Theory and text analysis. In W. C. Mann & S. A. Thompson (eds.) *Discourse description: Diverse linguistic analyses of a fund-raising text* (pp. 39–78). Amsterdam: John Benjamins.

Mann, W. C. & Thompson, S. A. 1988. Rhetorical Structure Theory: Toward a functional theory of text organization. *Text*, 8, 243–281.

Mann, W. C. & Thompson, S. A. 1992. *Discourse description: Diverse linguistic analyses of a fund-raising text*. Amsterdam; Philadelphia: John Benjamins.

Mehan, H. 1999. Oracular reasoning in a psychiatric exam. In A. Jaworski & N. Coupland (eds.) *The discourse reader* (pp. 559–575). London; New York: Routledge.

Message of the Vice Premier Li Lanqing to the Symposium on the World Health Day. 7 April 2001. Authors copy.

Metzger, T. A. 1981. Selfhood and authority in Neo-Confucian political culture. In A. Kleinman & T. Lin (eds.) *Normal and abnormal behaviour in Chinese culture* (pp. 7–28). Dordrecht; Boston: D. Reidel.

Miller, G. 1994. Towards ethnographies of institutional discourse: Proposal and suggestions. *Journal of Contemporary Ethnography*, 23 (3), 280–306.

Minas, I. H., Lambert, T. J. R., Kostov, S. & Boranga, G. 1996. *Mental health services for NESB immigrants: Transforming policy into practice*. Canberra: Australian Government Publishing Service.

Mishler, E. G. 1984. The *discourse of medicine: Dialectics of medical interviews*. Norwood: Ablex.

Multicultural Mental Health Australia. 2004. http://www.mmha.org.au

Mumby, D. K. & Clair, R. P. 1997. Organizational discourse. In T. A. Van Dijk (ed.) *Discourse studies: A multidisciplinary introduction, volume 2* (pp. 181–205). London: Sage Publications.

Ng, R. M. 2000. The influence of Confucianism on Chinese conceptions of power, authority, and the rule of law. In D. R. Heisey (ed.) *Chinese perspectives in rhetoric and communication* (pp. 45–56). Stamford: Ablex.

Ng, V. W. 1990. *Madness in late imperial China: From illness to deviance*. Norman and London: University of Oklahoma Press.

Noordman, L. G. M., Vonk, W. & Simons, W. H. G. 2000. Knowledge representation in the domain of economics. In L. Lundquist & R. J. Jarvella (eds.) *Language, text, and knowledge: Mental models of expert communication* (pp. 235–260). Berlin; New York: Mouton de Gruyter.

Nutbeam, D. & Harris, E. 1999. *Theory in a nutshell: A guide to health promotion theory*. Sydney: McGraw-Hill Book Co.

O'Donnell, L. 2002. Attack on zoo bears an 'intelligence test'. *The Australian*, Thursday February 28.

Pearson, V. 1991. The development of modern psychiatric services in China 1891–1949. *History of Psychiatry*, 2, 133–147.

Pearson, V. 1992. Law, rights and psychiatry in the People's Republic of China. *International Journal of Law and Psychiatry*, 15, 409–423.

Pearson, V. 1995a. Population policy and eugenics in China. *The British Journal of Psychiatry*, 167, 1–4.

Pearson, V. 1995b. Goods on which one loses: Women and mental health in China. *Social Science and Medicine*, 41 (8), 1159–1173.

Pearson, V. 1995c. *Mental health care in China: State policies, professional services and family responsibilities*. London: Gaskell.

Pearson, V. 1996. The Chinese equation in mental health policy and practice. *International Journal of Law and Psychiatry*, 19 (3/4), 437–458.

Pearson, V. & Phillips, M. 1994. Psychiatric social work and socialism: Problems and potential in China. *Social Work*, 39 (3), 280–287.

Pelsmaekers, K. & Geluykens, R. 1995. About (institutional) discourse. *Interface: Journal of Applied Linguistics*, 10 (1), 3–9.

Phillips, M. R. 1993. Strategies used by Chinese families coping with schizophrenia. In D. Davis & S. Harrell (eds.) *Chinese families in the post-Mao era* (pp. 277–306). Berkeley, CA: University of California Press

Phillips, M. R., Li, Y., Stroup, T. S. & Xin, L. 2000. Causes of schizophrenia reported by patients' family members in China. *The British Journal of Psychiatry*, 177, 20–25.

Phillips, M. R., Pearson, V., Li, F., Xu, M. and Yang, L. 2002. Stigma and expressed emotion: A study of people with schizophrenia and their family members in China. *British Journal of Psychiatry*, 181, 488–493.

Pu, S. 1916. *Strange stories from a Chinese studio* (translated and annotated by Giles, H. A.). Shanghai: Kelly & Walsh.

Qiu, J. L. 2000. Interpreting the Dengist rhetoric of building socialism with Chinese characteristics. In D. R. Heisey (ed.) *Chinese perspectives in rhetoric and communication* (pp. 249–280). Stamford: Ablex.

Ramsay, G. 1997. *Beijing review newstext: A comparative cross-cultural analysis of lexico-semantic and discourse structural features*. Unpublished doctoral dissertation. University of Queensland.

Ramsay, G. 2000. Linearity in rhetorical organisation: A comparative cross-cultural analysis of newstext from the People's Republic of China and Australia. *International Journal of Applied Linguistics*, 10 (2), 241–258.

Ramsay, G. 2001a. What are they getting at? Placement of important ideas in lengthy Chinese newstext: A contrastive analysis with Australian newstext. *Australian Review of Applied Linguistics*, 24 (2), 17–34.

Ramsay, G. 2001b. Rhetorical styles and newstexts: A contrastive analysis of rhetorical relations in Chinese and Australian news-journal text. *ASAA E-journal of Asian Linguistics and Language-teaching*, 1 (1), 1–22.

Ramsay, G. 2004a. (Mis)Communicating mental health: The discursive form of Chinese-language psychoeducational literature. In R. Cribb (ed.) *Asia examined: Proceedings of the 15th biennial conference of the ASAA, 2004, Canberra, Australia* (pp. 1–22). Canberra: Asian Studies Association of Australia (ASAA) & Research School of Pacific & Asian Studies (RSPAS), The Australian National University.

Ramsay, G. 2004b. The Chinese diaspora in Torres Strait: Cross-cultural connections and contentions on Thursday Island. In A. Shnukal, G. Ramsay & Y. Nagata (eds.) *Navigating boundaries: The Asian diaspora in Torres Strait* (pp. 53–79). Canberra: Pandanus.

Ran, M., Xiang, M., Simpson, P. & Chan, C. L. 2005. *Family-based mental health care in rural China*. Hong Kong: Hong Kong University Press.

Ran, M., et al. 2003. Effectiveness of psychoeducational intervention for rural Chinese families experiencing schizophrenia: A randomised control trial. *Social Psychiatry and Psychiatric Epidemiology*, 38 (2), 69–75.

Roberts, C. & Sarangi, S. 1999. Hybridity in gatekeeping discourse: Issues of practical relevance for the researcher. In S. Sarangi & C. Roberts (eds.) *Talk, work and institutional order: Discourse in medical, mediation and management settings* (pp. 473–504). New York: Mouton de Gruyter.

Rogers, W. S. 1991. *Explaining health and illness: An exploration of diversity*. New York; Sydney: Harvester Wheatsheaf.

Samovar, L. A. & Porter, R. E. 2001. *Communication between cultures*. Belmont, CA: Wadsworth/Thomson Learning.

Samovar, L. A. & Porter, R. E. 2003. An introduction and overview. In L. A. Samovar & R. E. Porter (eds.) *Intercultural communication: A reader* (pp. 6–17). Belmont, CA: Wadsworth/Thomson Learning.

Sanders, T. J. M., Spooren, W. P. M. & Noordman, L. G. M. 1992. Toward a taxonomy of coherence relations. *Discourse Processes*, 15, 1–35.

Sarangi, S. 1998. Institutional language. In J. L. Mey (ed.) *Concise encyclopaedia of pragmatics* (pp. 382–385). Oxford: Elsevier.

Sarangi, S. & Roberts, C. 1999. The dynamics of interactional and institutional orders in work-related settings. In S. Sarangi & C. Roberts (eds.) *Talk, work and institutional order: Discourse in medical, mediation and management settings* (pp. 1–60). New York: Mouton de Gruyter.

Sarangi, S. & Slembrouck, S. 1996. *Language, bureaucracy and social control*. London; New York: Longman.

Sarangi, S. & Slembrouck, S. 1997. Confrontational asymmetries in institutional discourse: A socio-pragmatic view of information exchange and face management. *Belgian Journal of Linguistics*, 11, 255–275.

Schiffrin, D. 1994. *Approaches to discourse*. Oxford: Blackwell.

Scollon, R. & Scollon, S. W. 1995. *Intercultural communication: A discourse approach*. Oxford; Cambridge, MA: Blackwell.

Selander, S., Troein, M., Finnegan, Jr, J. &. Råstam, L. 1997. The discursive formation of health: A study of printed health education material used in primary care. *Patient Education and Counselling*, 31, 181–189.

Sevigny, R., Yang, W., Zhang, R. & Marleau, J. D. 1999. Attitudes toward the mentally ill in a sample of professionals working in a psychiatric hospital in Beijing (China). *The International Journal of Social Psychiatry*, 45 (10), 41–45.

Steel, Z. P., McDonald, R. & Hornsey, J. 1995. NSW hospitalisation and community management of NESB migrants with mental disorders. In K. Kellehear, M. Teesson, J. Farhall, J. Peters, V. Miller & S. Robertson (eds.) *Prevention, partnership, integration: Meeting the challenges* (pp. 108–119). Balmain, NSW: Mental Health Services Conference Inc. of Australia & New Zealand.

Stuart-Smith, V. 2007. The hierarchical organization of text as conceptualized by Rhetorical Structure Theory: A systemic functional perspective. *Australian Journal of Linguistics*, 27 (1), 41–61.

Sue, S. & Morishima, J. K. 1982. *The mental health of Asian Americans*. San Francisco: Jossey-Bass Publishers.

Taboada, M. & Mann, W. C. 2006. Rhetorical Structure Theory: Looking back and moving ahead. *Discourse Studies*, 8 (3), 423–459.

Tabora, B. L. & Flaskerud, J. H. 1997. Mental health beliefs, practices, and knowledge of Chinese American immigrant women. *Issues in Mental Health Nursing*, 18, 173–189.

Tan, E. 1981. Culture-bound syndromes among overseas Chinese. In A. Kleinman & T. Lin (eds.) *Normal and abnormal behaviour in Chinese culture* (pp. 371–386). Dordrecht; Boston: D. Reidel.

Tannen, D. 1990. Discourse analysis: The excitement of diversity. *Text*, 10 (1/2), 109–111.

Thornborrow, J. 2002. *Power talk: Language and interaction in institutional discourse*. Harlow: Longman.

Ting-Toomey, S. 1999. *Communicating across cultures*. New York: Guilford Press.

Traphagan. J. W. 2000. *Taming oblivion: Aging bodies and the fear of senility in Japan*. New York: State University of New York Press.

Traphagan, J. W. 2004. *The practice of concern: Ritual, well-being, and aging in rural Japan*. Durham, NC: Carolina Academic Press.

Triandis, H. C. 2003. Culture and conflict. In L. A. Samovar & R. E. Porter (eds.) *Intercultural communication: A reader* (pp. 18–27). Belmont, CA: Wadsworth /Thomson Learning.

Tseng, W. 1973a. Concept of personality in Confucian thought. *Psychiatry*, 36, 191–202.

Tseng, W. 1973b. The development of psychiatric concepts in traditional Chinese medicine. *Archives of General Psychiatry*, 29, 569–575.

Tseng, W. 1986. Chinese psychiatry: Development and characteristics. In J. L. Cox (ed.) *Transcultural psychiatry* (pp. 274–290). London: Crown Helm.

Unschuld, P. U. 1985. *Medicine in China: A history of ideas*. Berkeley, CA: University of California Press.

Valle, E. 1998. Insider talk: The study of discourse in professional communities. *Anglicana Turkuensia*, 16, 111–126.

van Dijk, T. A. 1988. *News as discourse*. Hillsdale, NJ: Lawrence Erlbaum.

van Dijk, T. A. 1997. The study of discourse. In T. A. van Dijk (ed.) *Discourse studies: A multidisciplinary introduction, volume 1* (pp. 1–34). London: Sage.

Wang, J. 2002. Research on Chinese communication campaigns: A historical review. In W. Jia, X. Lu & D. R. Heisey (eds.) *Chinese communication theory and research: Reflections, new frontiers, and new directions* (pp. 131–146). London: Ablex.

White, M. 1995. *Re-authoring lives: Interviews and essays*. Adelaide: Dulwich Centre Publications.

Williams, B. & Healy, D. 2001. Perceptions of illness causation among new referrals to a community mental health team: "Explanatory model" or "exploratory map"? *Social Science and Medicine*, 53, 465–476.

Willig, C. 1999. Conclusion: Opportunities and limitations of 'applied discourse analysis'. In C. Willig (ed.) *Applied discourse analysis: Social and psychological interventions* (pp. 145–159). Buckingham: Open University Press.

Witte, K. & Morrison, K. 1995. Intercultural and cross-cultural health communication: Understanding people and motivating healthy behaviors. In R. L. Wiseman (ed.) *Intercultural communication theory* (pp. 216–246). Thousand Oaks: Sage Publications.

Wodak, R. 1996. *Disorders of discourse*. London; New York: Longman.

Wong, D. F. K. 2000. Stress factors and mental health of carers with relatives suffering from schizophrenia in Hong Kong: Implications for culturally sensitive practices. *British Journal of Social Work*, 30, 365–382.

Wood, L. A. & Kroger, R. O. 2000. *Doing discourse analysis: Methods for studying action in talk and text*. London: Sage Publications.

Xia, Z. & Zhang, M. 1981. History and present status of modern psychiatry in China. *Chinese Medical Journal*, 94 (5), 277–282.

Yan, H. 1985. Some psychological problems manifested by neurotic patients: Shanghai examples. In W. Tseng & D. Y. H. Wu (eds.) *Chinese culture and mental health* (pp. 325–338). London: Academic Press.

Yang, Y. K., Hsieh, H. H., Wu, A. C. C., Yeh, T. L. & Chen, C. C. 1999. Help-seeking behaviours in relatives of schizophrenics in Taiwan. *General hospital psychiatry*, 21, 303–309.

Yep, G. A. 2000. Explaining illness to Asian and Pacific Islander Americans: Culture, communication, and boundary regulation. In B. B. Whaley (ed.) *Explaining illness: Research, theory, and strategies* (pp. 281–296). Mahwah: Lawrence Erlbaum Associates.

Zhang, M., et al. 1993. Effectiveness of psychoeducation of relatives of schizophrenic patients: A prospective cohort study in five cities of China. *International Journal of Mental Health*, 22 (1), 47–59.

Zhang, X. 1988. *Half of man is women* (translated by Avery, M.). New York: W. W. Norton & Co.

Index

In the series *Discourse Approaches to Politics, Society and Culture* the following titles have been published thus far or are scheduled for publication:

32 **RAMSAY, Guy:** Shaping Minds. A discourse analysis of Chinese-language community mental health literature. 2008. ix, 149 pp.

31 **JOHNSTONE, Barbara and Christopher EISENHART (eds.):** Rhetoric in Detail. Discourse analyses of rhetorical talk and text. 2008. viii, 330 pp.

30 **POWERS, John H. and Xiaosui XIAO (eds.):** The Social Construction of SARS. Studies of a health communication crisis. 2008. vi, 242 pp.

29 **ACHUGAR, Mariana:** What We Remember. The construction of memory in military discourse. 2008. x, 246 pp.

28 **DOLÓN, Rosana and Júlia TODOLÍ (eds.):** Analysing Identities in Discourse. 2008. xi, 204 pp.

27 **VERDOOLAEGE, Annelies:** Reconciliation Discourse. The case of the Truth and Reconciliation Commission. 2008. xiii, 238 pp.

26 **MILLAR, Sharon and John WILSON (eds.):** The Discourse of Europe. Talk and text in everyday life. 2007. viii, 200 pp.

25 **AZUELOS-ATIAS, Sol:** A Pragmatic Analysis of Legal Proofs of Criminal Intent. 2007. x, 180 pp.

24 **HODGES, Adam and Chad NILEP (eds.):** Discourse, War and Terrorism. 2007. x, 248 pp.

23 **GOATLY, Andrew:** Washing the Brain – Metaphor and Hidden Ideology. 2007. xvii, 431 pp.

22 **LE, Elisabeth:** The Spiral of 'Anti-Other Rhetoric'. Discourses of identity and the international media echo. 2006. xii, 280 pp.

21 **MYHILL, John:** Language, Religion and National Identity in Europe and the Middle East. A historical study. 2006. ix, 300 pp.

20 **OMONIYI, Tope and Joshua A. FISHMAN (eds.):** Explorations in the Sociology of Language and Religion. 2006. viii, 347 pp.

19 **HAUSENDORF, Heiko and Alfons BORA (eds.):** Analysing Citizenship Talk. Social positioning in political and legal decision-making processes. 2006. viii, 368 pp.

18 **LASSEN, Inger, Jeanne STRUNCK and Torben VESTERGAARD (eds.):** Mediating Ideology in Text and Image. Ten critical studies. 2006. xii, 254 pp.

17 **SAUSSURE, Louis de and Peter SCHULZ (eds.):** Manipulation and Ideologies in the Twentieth Century. Discourse, language, mind. 2005. xvi, 312 pp.

16 **ERREYGERS, Guido and Geert JACOBS (eds.):** Language, Communication and the Economy. 2005. viii, 239 pp.

15 **BLACKLEDGE, Adrian:** Discourse and Power in a Multilingual World. 2005. x, 252 pp.

14 **DIJK, Teun A. van:** Racism and Discourse in Spain and Latin America. 2005. xii, 198 pp.

13 **WODAK, Ruth and Paul CHILTON (eds.):** A New Agenda in (Critical) Discourse Analysis. Theory, methodology and interdisciplinarity. 2005. xviii, 320 pp.

12 **GRILLO, Eric (ed.):** Power Without Domination. Dialogism and the empowering property of communication. 2005. xviii, 247 pp.

11 **MUNTIGL, Peter:** Narrative Counselling. Social and linguistic processes of change. 2004. x, 347 pp.

10 **BAYLEY, Paul (ed.):** Cross-Cultural Perspectives on Parliamentary Discourse. 2004. vi, 385 pp.

9 **RICHARDSON, John E.:** (Mis)Representing Islam. The racism and rhetoric of British broadsheet newspapers. 2004. vi, 277 pp.

8 **MARTIN, J.R. and Ruth WODAK (eds.):** Re/reading the past. Critical and functional perspectives on time and value. 2003. vi, 277 pp.

7 **ENSINK, Titus and Christoph SAUER (eds.):** The Art of Commemoration. Fifty years after the Warsaw Uprising. 2003. xii, 246 pp.

6 **DUNNE, Michele Durocher:** Democracy in Contemporary Egyptian Political Discourse. 2003. xii, 179 pp.

5 **THIESMEYER, Lynn (ed.):** Discourse and Silencing. Representation and the language of displacement. 2003. x, 316 pp.

4 **CHILTON, Paul and Christina SCHÄFFNER (eds.):** Politics as Text and Talk. Analytic approaches to political discourse. 2002. x, 246 pp.

3 **CHNG, Huang Hoon:** Separate and Unequal. Judicial rhetoric and women's rights. 2002. viii, 157 pp.

2 **LITOSSELITI, Lia and Jane SUNDERLAND (eds.):** Gender Identity and Discourse Analysis. 2002. viii, 336 pp.

1 **GELBER, Katharine:** Speaking Back. The free speech versus hate speech debate. 2002. xiv, 177 pp.